We do not know, we can only conjecture.
Science is not a system of certain knowledge,
but a system of conjectural hypotheses.

Karl Popper, Conjectures and Refutations, 1963

Exercise & Fibromyalgia
Theory, Research and Applications

Authors

Gianpiero Greco

Department of Translational Biomedicine and Neuroscience (DiBraiN)
University of Study of Bari "Aldo Moro"

Felice Festa

Department of Translational Biomedicine and Neuroscience (DiBraiN)
University of Study of Bari "Aldo Moro"

Vito Pugliese

Department of Translational Biomedicine and Neuroscience (DiBraiN)
University of Study of Bari "Aldo Moro"

Francesco Fischetti

Department of Translational Biomedicine and Neuroscience (DiBraiN)
University of Study of Bari "Aldo Moro"

CONTENTS

Authors' preface v

Chapter 1
THE FIBROMYALGIC SYNDROME

1.1 Clinical overview of the pathology	3
1.2 Epidemiology	5
1.3 Etiopathogenesis	7
1.4 Symptomatology...	11
1.5 Diagnosis	15
1.6 Prognosis and Treatment	20
1.7 Physical and motor disorders associated with Fibromyalgia Syndrome	27
1.8 Psychological aspects associated with Fibromyalgia Syndrome	29
References	35

Chapter 2
THE BENEFITS OF ADAPTED PHYSICAL ACTIVITY TO INDIVIDUALS WITH FIBROMYALGIA

2.1 The prescription of physical exercise as a non-pharmacological treatment	47

2.2 The effects of adapted physical activity on the pain neuromodulation process……....…………………… 51

2.3 The effects of different types of activities on physical abilities and functional status ……………………… 55

2.4 The effectiveness of body awareness therapies associated with fibromyalgia ……………………….. 60

References …………………………………………… 65

Chapter 3
PHYSICAL ACTIVITY AND PSYCHOPHYSICAL WELLBEING IN SUBJECTS WITH FIBROMYALGIA

3.1 Physical activity and psychological wellbeing……... 75

3.2 Effects of physical activity on pain, flexibility, balance and Quality of Life …………………………. 78

3.3 Targeted physical activity or nonspecific training? Comparison of the effects on Quality of Life…………………………………………………. 80

3.4 Effects of aquatic and dry land exercise on stress response ……………………………………….. 83

3.5 Physical fitness status in relation to depression, anxiety and Quality of Life …………………………. 88

References …………………………………………… 93

Chapter 4

SPECIFIC EXERCISE PROTOCOLS FOR FIBROMYALGIA SYNDROME

4.1 Aerobic activity protocols	105
4.2 Strength (Resistance) training protocols	113
4.3 Training protocols for flexibility and joint mobility ...	119
4.4 Combined or multicomponent training	125
4.5 Water training protocols	136
4.6 Pilates	144
4.7 Tai Chi	148
4.8 Dance as Movement Therapy	151
References	155

Chapter 5

GUIDELINES FOR EXERCISE PRESCRIPTION AND PRACTICAL APPLICATIONS

5.1 Training Programming: Theory and Applications	177
5.2 Exercise dosage in relation to FITT-VP training principles	195
5.2.1 Frequency	196
5.2.2 Intensity	197
5.2.3 Time	198
5.2.4 Type	199
5.2.5 Volume and Progression	200

5.3 Example of an exercise protocol adapted to subjects
    with Fibromyalgia …………………………………..   201
References …..……………………………………………..   211

Authors' preface

Fibromyalgia is a complex condition that affects millions of people worldwide. This book was born out of the need to provide a comprehensive and up-to-date guide on the prescription and administration of physical exercise, with a particular focus on the benefits of adapted physical activity as a "non-pharmacological" treatment.

In Chapter 1, we explored fibromyalgia syndrome in all its facets, from clinical framing to epidemiology, from etiopathogenesis to symptomatology, and finally to diagnosis, prognosis, and treatment. We also analyzed the physical and motor disorders, and the psychological aspects associated with the syndrome.

Chapter 2 was dedicated to the benefits of adapted physical activity for individuals with fibromyalgia. We discussed how exercise can be prescribed as a "non-pharmacological" treatment and its effects on the process of pain neuromodulation. We examined different types of exercise and their effectiveness on patients' physical abilities and functional status, as well as the importance of body awareness therapies.

In Chapter 3, we focused on the psychophysical well-being of individuals with fibromyalgia, exploring how physical activity can influence cognitive well-being, pain, flexibility, balance, and quality of life. We compared the effects of targeted physical activity versus non-specific training and analyzed the impact of exercise in water or on land on stress response.

Chapter 4 presents specific exercise protocols for fibromyalgia syndrome, including aerobic training, strength training, flexibility, and joint mobility. We also explored combined or multicomponent training, water training, Pilates, Tai Chi, and dance as movement therapy.

Finally, in Chapter 5, we provided practical guidelines for the prescription and administration of physical exercise, with particular attention to training programming and exercise dosage according to the FITT-VP principles. We concluded with an example of an exercise protocol adapted for individuals with fibromyalgia, with the availability of online videos showing the exercises to be performed via QR Code scanning.

We hope that this book can be a valuable resource for kinesiologists, physicians, physiotherapists, patients, and all those involved in the management of fibromyalgia. Our goal is to offer an in-depth understanding of the syndrome as well as the most effective "non-pharmacological" treatment par excellence, which is physical exercise, to improve the quality of life of patients.

Chapter 1
THE FIBROMYALGIC SYNDROME
by F. Fischetti, F. Festa, V. Pugliese, G. Greco

1.1 Clinical overview of the pathology

Fibromyalgia (FM) is a chronic syndrome characterized by widespread musculoskeletal pain and the presence of what are called tender points (TPs) (Wolfe et al., 1990).

The pathogenesis of FM is not completely known; however, the current concept sees FM as the result of an altered functioning of the central nervous system, which would determine the consequent amplification of the perception and transmission of pain (Gracely et al., 2002). FM is considered one of numerous relatively common "overlap" syndromes, characterized by chronic pain and fatigue, which are difficult to trace to other types of pathologies (Clauw, 2001). FM is more common in children of FM patients; there is, therefore, a familial component and in addition to this, environmental factors are critical in the onset of the disease. Genetic and environmental factors play a fundamental role in the pathogenesis of FM (Wolfe et al., 1990).

From a genetic point of view, it seems unlikely that the alteration of a single gene is responsible for the onset of FM symptoms; in fact, polymorphisms of various systems appear to be implicated, including the dopaminergic, catecholaminergic and serotoninergic systems. The pathology is very often "overlapped" (hence the term overlap) with other types of pathological conditions, the most widespread of which are chronic fatigue syndrome, irritable bowel syndrome and interstitial cystitis (Salaffi & Farah, 2019).

Clinical descriptions of what we now call FM have been reported since the mid-1800s. Originally, several terms were used to identify this condition, including "neurasthenia" and "muscular rheumatism". In 1904, Gowers created the term "fibrositis" (Gowers, 1904), which was mostly used until the 1970s and 1980s, when it was discovered that the etiology of this syndrome lay in the central nervous system (Mease, 2005). The term "fibromyalgia", introduced in 1976 by Hench, in fact, highlights the pain present in the muscles and fibrous connective structures (tendons-ligaments). In the classification of rheumatic diseases of the Italian Society of Rheumatology, FM is included among extra-articular rheumatism (Del Rosso & Maddaloni Bongi, 2015).

There are no specific instrumental tests capable of determining the presence of this pathology and there are no therapies either, in fact the treatments are often based on individual and peculiar approaches for the individual patient, given the variety of symptoms.

It also appears to be a complicated pathology to "endure", not only in physical terms and therefore about the link with the painful and tiring symptoms with which to live, but also above all in psychological terms, in fact, it is almost always experienced as an experience "invisible" and silent, little understood and often not recognized, because apparently, the patient has no obvious "signs" of suffering (tests and medical analyzes of normal diagnostic practice are normal) other than what he says he feels happening inside himself: Fibromyalgia sufferers are often considered an "imaginary patient" by doctors and family members (Perrot, 2019). From an epidemiological point of view, it is considered the third cause of chronic musculoskeletal pain, after lower back pain and osteoarthritis (Di Carlo et al., 2021).

1.2 Epidemiology

The prevalence of FM in the general population can be estimated on average at around 5%, in general, the prevalence varies in males between 0.1% and 3.9% and in women, between 2.5% and 10.5%, in women it increases with increasing age, up to 79 years; furthermore, a study conducted in Israel reports the presence of FM in children in 6.2% of cases (Buskila et al., 1993). In 2005 in Italy, Salaffi et al. conducted the MAPPING study to collect data on the prevalence of musculoskeletal diseases on a sample of the Italian population made up of 2,155 patients selected by General Practitioners. The prevalence of FM found was equal to 2.22%, which would identify 1,346,700 affected patients in our country, considering the ISTAT data on the population resident in Italy (Salaffi et al., 2005).

The study *"The Fell Study: Fibromyalgia Epidemiology European Large-scale survey"* of 2005 instead evaluated the prevalence of FM in the general population in some European states; the results indicate a prevalence of 4.3% in France (6.1% in women and 0.5% of men in a sample of 1000 inhabitants) and 6.1%

in Portugal (8.8% of women and 0.7% of men in a sample of 500 inhabitants) (Russell & Raphael, 2008).

From the analysis of data on prevalence in the general population, collected starting from the publication of the ACR classification criteria from 1990 until today, the presence of FM is observed in all ethnic groups studied and this does not seem limited to industrialized countries; however, the data varies greatly in different countries.

FM is often misunderstood and underestimated. It is reported that around 75% of people who suffer from it have not received an adequate diagnosis. Unfortunately, the age at which FM begins is decreasing; in fact, a 2021 study in "Pediatric Rheumatology" talks about juvenile primary fibromyalgia syndrome (JPFS) in younger children, the estimated prevalence varies from 1.2% to 6.2%, the age of onset is approximately 11.4 to 13.7 years, between 5 and 18 years.

Essentially, FM has proven to be the third most common musculoskeletal condition in terms of prevalence, after low back pain and osteoarthritis; however, it is predominantly a female disease, which means that it is mainly women who are involved, a fact that has been confirmed by various studies, which lead us to conclude that the average ratio between women and men is 3:1; the reasons for this disparity are many, women are predisposed from a physiological point of view to an alteration of the mechanisms of pain due to their biological processes which they undergo in the various phases of their life but they are also more inclined to suffer significantly the chronic psycho-physical stress linked to modern life, which sees them busy on multiple fronts (work, family); it should also be remembered that inflammatory and autoimmune diseases double or triple in females due to the effect of sexual hormones on the cells that regulate immune defences (Garritano, 2023).

1.3 Etiopathogenesis

The etiology and pathogenesis of FM are not yet completely clear, several factors appear to be involved such as dysfunction of the central and autonomic nervous system, neurotransmitters, hormones, the immune system, external stress factors, psychiatric aspects and many others (Bellato et al., 2012). Central sensitization is considered the main mechanism involved and is defined by the increased response to different stimulations, a response mediated by central nervous system signaling (Yunus, 1992). Central sensitization is the consequence of spontaneous nervous activity, enlarged receptive fields, and increased responses to stimuli transmitted by primary afferent fibers (Staud & Smitherman, 2002). An important phenomenon involved appears to be the "windup" which reflects the increased excitability of the neurons of the spinal cord and consists in the presence, following a painful stimulus, of subsequent stimuli of the same intensity which are perceived as stronger (Li et al., 1999); it is a phenomenon that occurs normally in all people (Mendell & Wall, 1965), but is altered and excessively perceived in fibromyalgia patients (Staud et al., 2001). These phenomena are an expression of neuroplasticity and are mediated mainly by N-methyl-D-aspartate (NMDA) receptors located in the postsynaptic membrane in the dorsal horn of the spinal cord (Dickenson, 1990; Staud & Domingo, 2001).

Another mechanism presumably involves the well-known descending pain inhibitory pathways, which modulate spinal cord responses to painful stimuli, these appear to be impaired in patients with FM, contributing to exacerbating central sensitization (Kosek & Hansson, 1997).

In addition to enhanced neuronal mechanisms, the activation of glial cells also appears to play an important role in the pathogenesis of FM, because these help to modulate pain transmission in the spinal cord. Activated by various painful stimuli, glial cells release pro-inflammatory cytokines, nitric oxide, prostaglandins and reactive oxygen species which stimulate and prolong spinal cord hyperexcitability (Watkins & Maier, 2005).

Furthermore, several neurotransmitters appear to be involved in central sensitization, in particular serotonin (5-HT) which appears to have a fundamental role in the modulation of pain (Dubner & Hargreaves, 1989), as well as being involved in the regulation of mood and sleep (Ressler & Nemeroff, 2000) and this could also explain the association between FM and sleep and mental disorders. This association creates a sort of vicious circle: patients affected by FM, as mentioned, often complain of sleep disturbances (Roizenblatt et al., 2001) and these, in turn, are probably involved in the pathogenesis itself (Bigatti et al., 2008), as a direct consequence of disturbed sleep determines a deficiency of GH and insulin-like growth factor 1 (IGF-1) (Cauter et al., 1998) and as these hormones are involved in the repair of muscle microtraumas, the repair of the same microtraumas, which would occur following the different muscular movements linked to the subjects' activity, would be ineffective, thus causing prolonged pain (Bennett et al., 1992).

Furthermore, the neuroendocrine system appears to be involved in the pathogenetic process of FM. This is because FM is considered a stress-related disorder, therefore it is easy to understand how the hypothalamic-pituitary-adrenal (HPA) axis may be involved (Crofford, 2002). Several studies have shown, that in fibromyalgia patients, high levels of cortisol, particularly in the evening, are associated with an interrupted circadian rhythm (Ferraccioli et al., 1990). Furthermore, the same patients showed high levels of adrenocorticotropic hormone (ACTH) both at baseline and in response to stress, most likely as a consequence of chronic hyposecretion of corticotropin-releasing hormone (CRH) (Griep et al., 1993).

In addition to glucocorticoids and growth factors, other types of hormones are also involved, for example, thyroid hormone levels are generally normal, although patients often show symptoms of hypothyroidism and there is some evidence to suggest an association with abnormal amounts of the thyrotropin-releasing hormone (TRH) (Garrison & Breeding, 2003).

Again, there is an association with the autonomic nervous system, in fact, various studies seem to confirm that in FM the sympathetic nervous system is persistently hyperactive, while it is hyporeactive in stressful situations. This could explain some clinical symptoms such as fatigue, morning stiffness, sleep disorders, anxiety, pseudo-Raynaud phenomenon, and intestinal irritability (Stisi et al., 2008).

Finally, we could identify some factors defined as triggers, such as some infections that seem to be able to induce FM, even if a direct causal relationship is not documented (Ablin et al., 2006). In particular, viruses such as HCV, HIV and Parvovirus could be involved (Rivera et al., 1997). An important role in this association could be played by cytokines and glial cells, which, for example, express receptors for bacteria and viruses (Gabuzda & Wang, 1999).

Physical trauma, vaccinations, and chemicals can also be triggers (Bell et al., 1998). However, it is worth remembering the results of Greenfield who did not notice any triggering factor in 72% of the patients included in his research (Greenfield et al., 1992). Therefore, we can state that it is not yet possible to determine a single cause associated with this type of pathology, but that several factors are involved in its etiology and pathogenesis process.

1.4 Symptomatology

FM presents no signs, but rather a series of symptoms (Salaffi et al., 2012); we can identify cardinal characteristics that include the most common symptoms as well as fundamental for a diagnosis according to the most recent criteria and other common characteristics that include widespread but less peculiar symptoms. The main symptoms are widespread pain, stiffness, fatigue and asthenia, intestinal/urogenital disorders, central nervous system and neurocognitive disorders and non-restful sleep (Salaffi et al., 2016), there are then others less frequent such as the sensation of swelling of the soft tissues, paresthesias/dysesthesias in the limbs, headache, neurovisceral and psychological disorders, sicca or Sjögren's syndrome (Cazzola et al., 2008). This protean symptomatology can be modulated by atmospheric variations and temperature. On cold, humid and rainy days the pain and stiffness are more intense, while most patients report a beneficial effect of the heat. Inactivity and hyperactivity aggravate the symptoms, which improve with moderate physical activity. The role of stress, whether physical or psychological, is known as a factor in worsening both pain and all the symptoms possibly associated with it. Chronic widespread pain that lasts for at least three months is the key symptom of FM and is described by the patient in various ways, such as a burning sensation, stiffness, and tension, like a cramp, a cut, a shock, a stab, or a burn. It causes disability to the patient, who, to reduce its intensity, reduces physical, daily and work activities. The intensity of the pain of patients with FM was found to be higher than that of patients with rheumatoid arthritis and more disabling than other rheumatic diseases, as it is accompanied by greater psychological distress. The patient describes the pain with expressions such as "it hurts everywhere", or "everywhere you touch me, it hurts". It is a "central" pain that does not have a constant location and entity but migrates and can increase or decrease throughout the day (Salaffi et al., 2005). Patients perceive even usually harmless external stimuli, such as touch or wearing clothes, as painful. These characteristics can be classified as allodynia (perception of pain following a harmless stimulus) and hyperalgesia (increased sensitivity to pain, which occurs in the case of mild stimuli) (Cazzola et al., 2014). These characteristics are specific to "central pain", different from those of "peripheral pain" of a mechanical or inflammatory nature, in which both the localization and intensity are much more constant (Salaffi et al., 2018).

The pain is very frequently accompanied by stiffness (84-91% of cases), generally lasting less than 30 minutes, generalized or localized to the trunk, which occurs mainly upon awakening (morning stiffness) or following prolonged maintenance of the same position, but also in the evening after a working day;

regarding fatigue and asthenia (these are symptoms reported by 75/90% of patients with FM), they can often become predominant and be perceived as prevalent compared to painful symptoms. Reduced resistance to fatigue, tiredness and weakness can worsen to the point of extreme difficulty carrying out any movement (bedridden patients). The relevant consequences are the strong difficulty in carrying out normal daily activities but also affect the intellectual, emotional and psychological spheres. Among the most common symptoms we also have headaches, especially nuchal, and muscle tension, but also temporal, supraorbital, maxillary or mandibular headaches, or migraines, sometimes the headache is widespread throughout the scalp, simple touching it dramatically exacerbates the pain (Salaffi & Farah, 2019).

Neurocognitive disorders are also often present in patients with FM, which include the loss of concentration and the ability to fix short-term memory, slowed gestures, the inability to carry out several tasks at the same time, easy distraction and cognitive overload. Gastrointestinal disorders such as digestive difficulties, abdominal pain, alternating constipation and diarrhea, which take the form of "irritable bowel syndrome" (Cassisi et al., 2008), are commonly observed in patients with FM.

In 60% of fibromyalgia patients there are mood disorders such as anxiety and depression, but also hypochondria and panic attacks, their presence has led to interpreting the disease as psychosomatic. Only 30-40% of patients experience a significant psychological disorder. The most frequent is the state of anxiety, reported in 13-64% of cases, but numerous studies have ruled out that FM could represent a particular form of hypochondriasis. Often there is a "secondary depression", reactive to the general deterioration of the state of health. "Catastrophization" represents a common cognitive style present during FM, which involves an exaggerated amplification of emotional aspects, with a pessimistic vision, which makes the pain considered intolerable (Lee et al., 2018).

Sleep disorders are almost constant (80-90% of cases) in fibromyalgia patients and lead to an accentuation of pain and asthenia upon awakening. In addition to the difficulty falling asleep, the patient has sleep disturbed by frequent nocturnal awakenings and non-restorative (Choy et al., 2015).

Furthermore, sensitivity disorders can occur, especially in terms of sight, touch, hearing and smell and are essentially represented by excessive sensitivity to external stimulations, whereby stimuli usually considered "comfortable" can be perceived as particularly intense. Visual blurring, and difficulty focusing when carrying out precision activities or while driving motor vehicles, often cause nausea and dizziness. Balance disorders consist of a sensation of instability and staggering, especially when standing for a long time. The causes can be traced back to visual disturbances, persistent contracture of the neck muscles, and neuro-mediated hypotension characterized by a feeling of fainting, nausea, dizziness, and visual blurring. Perception disorders are constant, such as paresthesias with a non-metameric distribution, in the form of tingling spread throughout the body or limited to a hemisome or the limbs, sensation of needle pricks, numbness or "falling asleep" of a limb, sensation of swelling in the hands and feet, abnormal sensations of cold or intense heat spread throughout the body or limbs (Salaffi & Sarzi-Puttini, 2012).

1.5 Diagnosis

FM, unlike almost all pathologies that characterize modern society, which are diagnosed thanks to blood chemistry and instrumental tests and/or the presence of specific symptoms, is not easily diagnosed; the importance of an early diagnosis that avoids not only the worsening of the symptoms of FM but also the establishment of vicious cycles such as pain-mood disorders, pain-immobility, which make management complex, is understandable. The combination of the numerous clinical manifestations and the severity of each individual symptom presents an extreme variability from patient to patient, which makes the early recognition of FM problematic (Bennett et al., 2010); although it is a clinical condition that has been known for some time, it has only recently received a scientific definition and formal recognition. The first criteria for the classification of FM were proposed in 1990 by the American College of Rheumatology (ACR) (Salaffi et al., 2012) and in 1992 the World Health Organization recognized fibromyalgia syndrome as a pathology (Copenhagen Declaration), with inclusion in the International Statistical Classification of Diseases and Related Health Problems (ICD) (January 1993): code "M79.0: Non-specific rheumatism". The ACR classification criteria formulated in 1990 require the presence of widespread musculoskeletal pain persisting for over three months and the positivity of at least 11 of the 18 Tender Points (TPs), evoked by acupressure induced by a pressure of 4 kg/cm2 or using a pressure algometer positioned in coded locations (Wolfe et al., 1990).

Figure 1.1 shows the anatomical locations of the 18 tender points used in the ACR classification criteria for the diagnosis of FM.

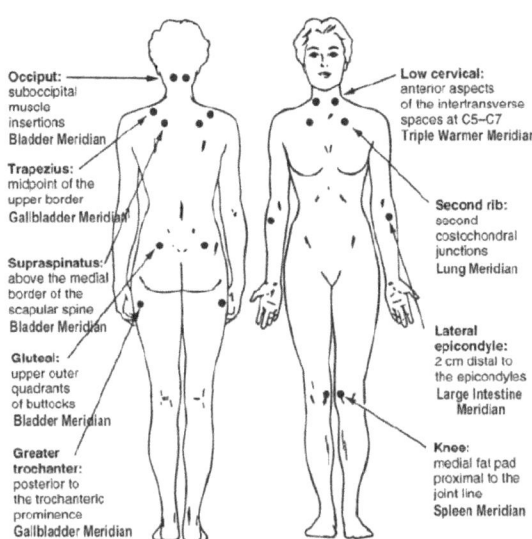

Figure 1.1 - Anatomical locations of "tender points" in fibromyalgia (Leskowitz, 2008).

The evaluation of Tender Points was often carried out imprecisely or incorrectly. The search for these points also requires a certain amount of manual skill, so incorrect identification of the areas or the application of excessive force can lead to diagnostic errors. Furthermore, the 1990 ACR criteria do not consider other symptoms such as asthenia, rigidity, changes in sleep, mood and neurological symptoms present in more than half of patients. The observation that the same patient can meet the criteria for several different syndromes has led many rheumatologists to question not only the specificity of the 1990 ACR criteria but the very existence of FM as a distinct nosological entity (Sarzi-Puttini et al., 2018). Given the numerous doubts raised by the scientific community regarding the usefulness of formulating the diagnosis of FM through Tender Points research, in 2010, new classification criteria were formulated by the American College of Rheumatology (ACR); the new classification criteria proposed the combination of the following two main variables Widespread Pain Index (WPI) and Symptom Severity Score (SSS).

Widespread Pain Index (WPI) includes a checklist of 19 areas of the body and the patient is invited to count the specific areas in which he felt pain in the week preceding the completion of the questionnaire, giving each a score equal to 1, with a total score between 0 and 19.

Symptom Severity Score (SSS) originates from the sum of the scores of somatic symptoms, non-restorative sleep, cognitive symptoms, and fatigue on a scale of 0-12. The SSS scale alone provides a measure of the severity of FM symptoms. For each of the three symptoms, the degree of severity perceived by the patient during the last week is indicated (Wolfe et al., 2010).

Combining the WPI and SSS scales led to the new definition of FM. To meet these classification criteria the patient must meet the following 3 conditions: widespread pain index (WPI) ≥7 and symptom severity scale (SS) score ≥5 or WPI between 3 and 6 and scale score for SS ≥9; symptoms present with the same intensity and persistent for at least 3 months; absence of concomitant clinical conditions that could motivate the pain.

The new criteria standardize diagnosis based on symptoms so that all doctors use the same procedure. The clinical diagnosis, although simpler, remains, however, essentially based on the doctor's subjective assessment of the extent and severity of the patient's somatic symptoms, not allowing self-assessment of the symptoms by the patient. For this reason, in 2011, a modification of the ACR 2010 criteria was proposed, in which the areas of pain and the presence/absence of 3 symptoms in SSS (headache, abdominal pain or cramps and depressive symptoms) are self-assessed by the patient (Wolfe et al., 2011). In 2013, a further modification was proposed which increased the areas of pain localization, and the number of symptoms, improving its specificity, regardless of the coexistence of another painful condition (Bennett et al., 2014). It is important to underline, however, that both the 2010 criteria and the subsequent versions of 2011 and 2013, although easier and quicker to perform, do not require the finding of objective clinical signs, an essential element in the diagnostic process of such a pathology. as complex as FM. In 2016, a further revision of the criteria was proposed by the ACR based on the integration of the criteria formulated in 2010 (*physician-based*) with the self-administered criteria (*self-report*) proposed and validated in 2011. The diagnosis of FM must be considered valid, regardless of other diagnoses or concomitant diseases and, in any case, does not exclude the presence of other clinically relevant disorders.

Recently, in 2018, thanks to the partnership between ACTTION (Analgesic, Anesthetic, and Addiction Clinical Trial Translations Innovations Opportunities and Networks) with the US Food and Drug Administration (FDA) and the American Pain Society (APS), the ACTTION-APS Pain Taxonomy (AAPT) to develop simplified diagnostic criteria for FM. These criteria, as for the previous ones, are exclusively based on clinical symptoms, do not include the counting of Tender Points and require the persistence of chronic pain (for at least 3 months) in 6 or more body areas, of the 9 identified locations, in association with coexistence of moderate or severe sleep or fatigue disorders; the AAPT criteria are, at the moment, considered poorly performing, compared to the criteria formulated in 2016 and are associated with a high rate of "false positives" (Wolfe, 2019).

1.6 Prognosis and Treatment

The overall approach to treating FM should focus on improving quality of life and managing symptoms, as it is impossible to completely recover from the condition (Bair & Krebs, 2020). To achieve these goals, the guidelines recommend an individualized and multimodal therapeutic approach. At the beginning of treatment, each patient should receive information about their diagnosis, especially the underlying pathophysiology and treatment options, including an introduction and discussion of self-management strategies (Bair & Krebs, 2020). These strategies may include stress management, information on sleep hygiene rules, a balanced diet, regular physical activity including aerobic exercise, weight reduction, pacing of activities and maintaining an overall healthy lifestyle. Coexisting conditions, such as sleep disorders and major depressive disorder, should be identified early and treated concurrently (Bair & Krebs, 2020). When initiating treatments, patients should be advised of reasonable expectations of benefit, reassessment should be scheduled, and treatments should be discontinued if benefits are not evident after a reasonable trial period. Because no single treatment improves function and minimizes all symptoms, a combination of treatments will likely be necessary. Treatment guidelines recommend that the initial management of patients with FM can and should be carried out in the primary care setting (Fitzcharles et al., 2013).

The role of psychological and behavioral therapies (CBT) has been identified, providing small incremental benefits over control interventions in relieving pain, improving mood and reducing disability at the end of treatment and during long-term follow-up. term (Bernardy et al., 2013). Furthermore, psychological interventions can be effective in improving physical function, pain, and mood compared to usual care (Theadom et al., 2015). Although treatment benefits are modest, psychological therapies are clearly safer than pharmacological agents and are likely associated with lower costs. Potential barriers to psychological therapies include limited access to therapists with experience managing patients with FM or patients' reluctance to consult a mental health provider (Friesen et al., 2017). To improve access, smartphone-based and technology-delivered interventions have been developed and tested. For example, an internet-based self-management program and an internet-delivered CBT course both resulted in benefits (reduced pain, improved depression, and increased satisfaction) for patients with FM (Friesen et al., 2017). The importance and use of psychological and behavioral therapies should therefore be emphasized, given their effectiveness, safety and cost advantages.

All FM patients should be educated about the importance of sleep in moderating pain, fatigue, and cognitive symptoms. Patients should also be evaluated for the presence of sleep disorders, including sleep apnea and insomnia, because specific therapies as well as information on sleep hygiene are needed for those who suffer from these disorders (Qaseem et al., 2016). For patients with insomnia, CBT for insomnia (CBT-I) is the first-line treatment (Qaseem et al., 2016), while the use of over-the-counter or prescription sedative hypnotics should generally be avoided.

Regarding pharmacological treatment, however, to alleviate the symptoms of FM, different classes of drugs can be tried. Tricyclic antidepressants (TCAs) have been used in clinical practice for decades as initial therapy (O'Malley et al., 2000). Potential adverse effects can be minimized by starting with low doses of amitriptyline at night and slowly increasing doses. Other TCAs, such as nortriptyline and desipramine, could be tried, but these are not as well studied (Moore et al., 2014).

In patients who are contraindicated, unresponsive, or have intolerable side effects to TCAs, a serotonin-norepinephrine reuptake inhibitor (SNRI) may be considered. SNRIs, particularly duloxetine and milnacipran, have been shown to provide benefits in several studies (Moore et al., 2014). Although few long-term studies exist on SNRIs, duloxetine is safe and effective and may be a good choice in patients with severe fatigue or comorbid depression (Murakami et al., 2017). Furthermore, gabapentinoids (gabapentin and pregabalin) have also been shown to benefit FM patients (Moore et al., 2014), however, a recent systematic review concluded that there is insufficient evidence to support or refute the hypothesis that Gabapentin reduces pain in FM (Cooper et al., 2017). Simple analgesics, such as paracetamol and non-steroidal anti-inflammatory drugs, are often prescribed as adjunctive therapy to relieve pain (Derry et al., 2017), but have not been shown to be effective in FM.

Research also suggests that patients with FM have alterations in the endogenous opioid system and may also have improved pain when treated with low doses of the opioid antagonist naltrexone (Younger et al., 2013). Although opioids are unlikely to benefit FM patients, epidemiological studies indicate that long-term opioid therapy is commonly prescribed for them (Goldenberg et al., 2016).

Randomized, controlled trials of manual acupuncture and electroacupuncture suggest benefits for pain, fatigue, and well-being, although the studies are small and mostly short-term (Lauche et al., 2015). For manual therapies, such as chiropractic manipulation, massage and myofascial release, the evidence is very limited and does not suggest a substantial benefit in FM (Lauche et al., 2015).

About the role of dietary modifications in the treatment or prevention of flare-ups, despite significant interest among patients in "anti-inflammatory" and other popular diets, evidence to support any nutritional intervention particular to FM is lacking. A recent review found that 7 clinical trials of different diets (low-calorie, vegetarian, and low-FODMAP) had similar positive results, but all trials were small and had substantial risk of bias (Silva et al., 2019). Given the low quality of evidence, appropriate dietary guidance for patients with FM may be similar to that for the general population, including calorie reduction for weight loss when appropriate.

FM patients should be followed regularly for assessment of symptom severity and functioning, treatment response, adherence, and adverse effects (Fitzcharles et al., 2013). The number of annual visits should be adjusted based on disease severity at diagnosis, comorbidity burden, symptom severity, changes in treatment plan, adverse effects of treatment, and patient preferences. An ideal approach to chronic disease management requires time to find the most effective treatment or combination of treatments for each patient (Fitzcharles et al., 2013). Evaluating the response to different treatments in a stepwise manner requires trials and reevaluations. More frequent outpatient visits may be needed at diagnosis and after starting new treatments (Fitzcharles et al., 2013), helping to manage flare-ups, encourage patients with suboptimal adherence, support patients who are overwhelmed by their condition, provide ongoing education, and emphasize self-management strategies. Furthermore, greater outpatient commitment has been found to protect FM patients from suicide (McKernan et al., 2019).

Beyond this, a pillar of treatment appears to be represented by active non-pharmacological therapies (supervised and gradual exercise programs and cognitive behavioral interventions) (Macfarlane et al., 2017; Rahman et al., 2014). Although medications are often used first due to practice models that rely more on pharmacological management than nonpharmacological therapies, they are associated with adverse effects and clinical trials show modest benefits in patients (Bair & Krebs, 2020).

The last fundamental element is patient education, in fact, it is an important component to validate the experience of the disease, reduce anxiety related to symptoms and provide motivation for self-management and recommended therapies. To optimize the likelihood of treatment success, clinicians should provide ongoing support for lifestyle changes and participation in active nonpharmacological therapies (Bair & Krebs, 2020). Patients should be informed that symptom exacerbations (flare-ups) are common and should be taught several possible strategies (keeping a symptom log and writing down triggers, reducing stress, using relaxation exercises, engaging in pleasant activities, and resting) to prevent and manage them. Treatment of FM should therefore be multimodal and multidisciplinary, using a combination of physical, behavioral and pharmacological therapies (Bair & Krebs, 2020).

Symptoms of FM can begin after physical trauma, surgery, infection, or significant psychological stress. In other cases, symptoms develop gradually and accumulate over time, without a single triggering event. Most patients will continue to have persistent pain and fatigue with intermittent fluctuations in symptoms over time (Bair & Krebs, 2020). Some studies have shown that pain, fatigue, sleep disturbances, anxiety and depression were essentially unchanged during 8 years of follow-up among patients visited in 6 different centers (Wolfe et al., 1997). In a more recent observational study, only 1 in 4 patients followed for up to 11 years reported at least moderate improvement in pain (Walitt et al., 2011). In contrast, some research has found that only 35% of patients still had widespread pain 2 years after the initial evaluation (Fitzcharles et al., 2003).

Of note, patients treated by community primary care physicians have a better prognosis than those seen in referral centers. Another important element linked to prognosis appears to be determined by work disability, which is common in patients with FM. 41.5% of patients with FM received Social Security disability compared to 36.8% and 23.7% of those with rheumatoid arthritis and osteoarthritis, respectively (Wolfe et al., 2014). The prognosis, therefore, is related to certain demographic, behavioral and psychological factors. Female sex, low socioeconomic status and unemployment status are associated with worse outcomes (Reisine et al., 2008). Other important prognostic factors include depression, history of abuse, catastrophizing, excessive somatic worry, and obesity (Mundal et al., 2014). Patients with FM have an increased risk of suicide and should therefore be monitored for symptoms of depression (Dreyer et al., 2010).

1.7 Physical and motor disorders associated with Fibromyalgia Syndrome

The presence of the main symptom of FM, i.e. musculoskeletal pain, determines in most cases the onset of some disorders related to the musculoskeletal system. However, pain does not appear to be the only factor linked to this phenomenon of functional disorder, in fact research has shown that cognitive factors (such as beliefs, evaluations and expectations) play an important role in determining adaptation to symptoms in patients with chronic pain (Turk & Okifuji, 2002). As has been observed in many chronic pain syndromes, maladaptive thoughts and information processing appear to be closely associated with the functional limitations observed in FM (Hassett et al., 2000). In fact, patients with FM who report a high fear of pain and physical activity also report greater disability. Several studies have shown that fear of pain and activity in patients with chronic pain is associated with poor physical performance, even when controlling for the pathology from a symptomatic point of view (Crombez et al., 1999) which appear to be linked to daily life. These findings are consistent with additional previous studies that have found that a specific fear of pain is a better predictor of disability than biomedical variables (symptoms) or even the severity and duration of the pain itself (Waddell et al., 1993). A plausible way to interpret this relationship is to hypothesize that fear of pain and activity instigates the avoidance of the activity itself and therefore increases the risk of physical deconditioning and the deconditioning, in turn, would contribute to the individual's disability (Waddell et al., 1993). The combination therefore of these factors, pain and cognitive elements associated with the pathology, tends to lead to what appears to be an almost total abandonment of any form of movement that goes beyond daily activities, sometimes even including them (Waddell et al., 1993). This is further associated with the stabilization of a very low functional motor level, which determines a condition of slight hypertonia, in some cases, walking disorders and above all persistent fatigue even during simple activities (Waddell et al., 1993).

The low level of physical activity is presumably explained by the habit of avoiding the aggravation of pain and fatigue (Vlaeyen et al., 2001), which consequently results in a sedentary lifestyle and deconditioned muscles (Vlaeyen et al., 1995) . A low level of physical activity may also be related to poor motor control and slower movement speed (Turk et al., 2004).

Another persistent element from a physical point of view, linked to fibromyalgia syndrome, is the onset of fatigue which occurs very rapidly when carrying out activities even with low cardiovascular commitment. Fatigue, as perceived and reported in the patient with FM, is the result of at least two different but interconnected mechanisms: a failure of central motor control and the remodeling of muscle fibers (Casale et al., 2009). These two aspects can be described differently in the clinic with a range of clinical and neurophysiological pictures ranging from a feeling of disabling fatigue but with preservation of the muscular fibrous composition, to a minimal sensation of tiredness associated with evident signs of muscular deconditioning. Fibromyalgia muscle has the same pattern of type I fibers that is recorded in healthy, deconditioned elderly individuals and can be counteracted by physical activity adapted to the type of fibers involved (Casale et al., 2003).

In conclusion, FM appears to be a very disabling pathology in terms of physical performance, even linked to simple activities; this occurs due to a series of factors that come together to determine a lowering of the individual's functional level and a worsening of his aerobic capacity.

1.8 Psychological aspects associated with Fibromyalgia Syndrome

In FM patients, in addition to the sensory component, the affective and cognitive aspects that accompany the pain are also fundamental; the psychological variables involved in the central processing of the painful stimulus, i.e. involved in the transition from the nociceptive stimulus to the perception of pain, are numerous, these seem to determine the different modulation of the pain threshold and the wide variety of behaviors in response to it and allow to explain the lack of congruence between the real existing damage and the persistence of the pain itself (Conversano & Marchi, 2018).

The variables that seem to play a central role in the establishment and chronicity of a painful condition such as FM are beliefs and attributions of meaning peculiar to the experience of pain, mood tone, emotional responses, coping strategies, variables of personality; in conditions of chronic pain the cognitive aspects contribute substantially to the characteristics of the pain, to the meaning that the person attributes and to the resulting behavioral response; based on certain beliefs and evaluations regarding the pain the person can decide to ignore it by continuing to work and socialize or leave their activities and take on the sick role. This evaluation, influencing how people respond to pain, takes on significant importance in the impact that FM can have on the life of the person affected by it. Incorrect beliefs regarding the origin of pain and its inevitability and the tendency towards self-blame are associated with greater intensity in the perception of pain, lower compliance with treatment and a greater level of stress (Conversano & Marchi, 2018).

Among the cognitive variables that play an important role in the perception of pain and its management are the low self-efficacy perceived in pain control, i.e. the belief in one's poor ability to face and manage pain, and the perception of loss of control over the same, which contributes to the presence of depressive symptoms, reduced self-esteem, poor adherence to therapies and the implementation of non-adaptive coping strategies, among which there is often a significant reduction in daily activities. Another cognitive aspect involved in FM is catastrophism, among the variables most frequently found in fibromyalgia patients, as well as the target of a possible therapeutic path. It seems to be the characteristic that most predicts the intensity of perceived pain, the increased sensitivity to it, the limitations in daily and work activities, the consumption of analgesics and the decrease in mobility and muscle strength over time. Catastrophizing is a cognitive process characterized by negative worries and ruminations about pain, which lead the patient to focus attention on painful stimuli. The amount of attention a person pays to a painful sensation can influence the intensity of its perception. When the focus of attention is directed towards other aspects of life, the painful experience is in fact experienced as less annoying (Hassett et al., 2000).

Regarding the psychological variables that influence the perception of pain, an important role is played by emotions. Emotions such as anger, frustration and fear are related to changes in the activity of the autonomic nervous system and appear to contribute to an increase in symptoms. Anger can play a central role in maintaining the disorder, causing an increase in muscle tension which, in turn, leads to an increase in pain. Anger is a common reaction in fibromyalgia patients, partly due to the limitations that pain creates in their lives, partly due to the frequent reactions of family members and some doctors who, by pointing them out as "imaginary patients", increase their experiences of loneliness, isolation and absence of hope. The relationship between pain and emotional state is bidirectional, the emotional state influencing the perception of pain and vice versa (Conversano & Marchi, 2018; Ressler & Nemeroff, 2000).

Mood also plays an important role in the onset and maintenance of chronic pain: it is common to observe mood disorders in fibromyalgia patients, mostly relating to the depressive spectrum. The presence of depression is associated with greater physical symptoms and greater persistence of pain. The mutual interaction between FM and depression worsens the course, duration and severity of symptoms and quality of life. The still unresolved question is whether it is depressive symptoms that precede FM, whether it is the opposite or whether they are both the expression of a common underlying psychopathological core (Ressler & Nemeroff, 2000).

Regarding anxiety, high levels of anxious symptoms and stress would lead to a lowering of the pain threshold and dysfunctional coping strategies. Fibromyalgia patients generally present very high levels of anxiety, so much so that it is assumed that chronic anxiety causes hyperactivation of the sympathetic system (Ressler & Nemeroff, 2000).

FM is also generally considered to be a stress-related pathology: an association has been found between the diagnosis of FM and a stressful life event preceding the diagnosis. In addition to the worsening of symptoms in conjunction with stressful events, these patients frequently present a life history characterized by negative events, often of a traumatic nature (Rosenbaum et al., 2015; Stubbs et al., 2017).

The meaning attributed to pain in the context of personal experience helps to determine the coping strategies used, i.e. the behavioral methods with which the subject deals with their condition. Subjects with a high sense of self-efficacy tend to use active coping strategies oriented towards solving the problem; subjects with a low sense of self-efficacy abandon the use of active coping strategies early because they anticipate failure. The adoption of this dysfunctional style in dealing with one's situation is defined as anomalous illness behavior, understood as "a mode of poor learning in perceiving, evaluating and acting in relation to one's state of health" (Conversano & Marchi, 2018).

Patients suffering from chronic pain tend to implement strategies aimed at controlling pain in an attempt to reduce or eliminate it. Often, in addition to taking drugs in acute moments, they take painkillers before the pain arises, showing an excessive and constant need to want to control their symptoms, as well as excessive attention to the symptoms and constant monitoring of the physiological bodily sensations. Furthermore, still, in an attempt to control it, some patients tend to avoid situations that could trigger pain, thus implementing avoidance strategies: not only are they more likely to abandon work and various domestic activities, but also recreational ones, taking the sick role (Conversano & Marchi, 2018).

The association between FM and psychiatric disorders, especially of a depressive and anxious nature, has been known for some time; Major depression has been studied with particular attention both for its frequency throughout the life of subjects with FM, estimated at around 70%, and for its negative impact on pain tolerance and the patient's social and work functioning. The diagnosis of major depression is particularly complex in fibromyalgia subjects, as many of the characteristic symptoms of FM are also common to the depressive episode; in particular, common symptoms are disturbed and unrestful sleep, concentration difficulties, persistent tiredness and feelings of inadequacy and guilt, it is, therefore, necessary to look for symptoms, such as lack of interest and pleasure in activities previously cultivated with satisfaction, which are elements characteristic of depression and not of FM. Such a high presence of depression in subjects affected by FM, according to a first hypothesis, can be explained by the fact that depression appears as a secondary disorder to the debilitating and chronic symptoms produced by FM. However, the evidence regarding a higher frequency of depressive pathology in FM than that observable in diseases with a severe prognosis calls into question its validity (Conversano & Marchi, 2018; Ressler & Nemeroff, 2000).

References

Ablin, J. N., Shoenfeld, Y., & Buskila, D. (2006). Fibromyalgia, infection and vaccination: Two more parts in the etiological puzzle. *Journal of Autoimmunity, 27*(3), 145–152.

Bair, M. J., & Krebs, E. E. (2020). Fibromyalgia. *Annals of Internal Medicine, 172*(5), ITC33–ITC48.

Bell, I. R., Baldwin, C. M., & Schwartz, G. E. (1998). Illness from low levels of environmental chemicals: Relevance to chronic fatigue syndrome and fibromyalgia. *The American journal of medicine, 105*(3), 74S-82S.

Bellato, E., Marini, E., Castoldi, F., Barbasetti, N., Mattei, L., Bonasia, D. E., & Blonna, D. (2012). Fibromyalgia syndrome: Etiology, pathogenesis, diagnosis, and treatment. *Pain research and treatment, 2012*.

Bennett, R. M., Clark, S. R., Campbell, S. M., & Burckhardt, C. S. (1992). Low levels of somatomedin C in patients with the fibromyalgia syndrome. A possible link between sleep and muscle pain. *Arthritis & Rheumatism: Official Journal of the American College of Rheumatology, 35*(10), 1113–1116.

Bennett, R. M., Friend, R., Marcus, D., Bernstein, C., Han, B. K., Yachoui, R., ... & Jones, K. D. (2014). Criteria for the diagnosis of fibromyalgia: validation of the modified 2010 preliminary American College of Rheumatology criteria and the development of alternative criteria. *Arthritis care & research, 66*(9), 1364-1373.

Bennett, R. M., Russell, J., Cappelleri, J. C., Bushmakin, A. G., Zlateva, G., & Sadosky, A. (2010). Identification of symptom and functional domains that fibromyalgia patients would like to see improved: a cluster analysis. *BMC Musculoskeletal Disorders, 11*, 1-10.

Bernardy, K., Klose, P., Busch, A. J., Choy, E. H., & Häuser, W. (2013). Cognitive behavioural therapies for fibromyalgia. *Cochrane Database of Systematic Reviews, 9*.

Bigatti, S. M., Hernandez, A. M., Cronan, T. A., & Rand, K. L. (2008). Sleep disturbances in fibromyalgia syndrome: Relationship to pain and depression. *Arthritis Care & Research: Official Journal of the American College of Rheumatology, 59*(7), 961–967.

Buskila, D., Press, J., Gedalia, A., Klein, M., Neumann, L., Boehm, R., & Sukenik, S. (1993). Assessment of nonarticular tenderness and prevalence of fibromyalgia in children. *The Journal of rheumatology*, *20*(2), 368-370.

Casale, R., Rainoldi, A., Nilsson, J., & Bellotti, P. (2003). Can continuous physical training counteract aging effect on myoelectric fatigue? A surface electromyography study application. *Archives of physical medicine and rehabilitation*, *84*(4), 513–517.

Casale, R., Sarzi-Puttini, P., Atzeni, F., Gazzoni, M., Buskila, D., & Rainoldi, A. (2009). Central motor control failure in fibromyalgia: A surface electromyography study. *BMC Musculoskeletal Disorders*, *10*(1), 78. https://doi.org/10.1186/1471-2474-10-78

Cassisi, G., Sarzi-Puttini, P., Alciati, A., Casale, R., Bazzichi, L., Carignola, R., ... & Atzeni, F. (2008). Symptoms and signs in fibromyalgia syndrome. *Reumatismo*, *60*(s1), 15-24.

Cauter, E. V., Plat, L., & Copinschi, G. (1998). Interrelations between sleep and the somatotropic axis. *Sleep*, *21*(6), 553–566.

Cazzola, M., Atzeni, F., Boccassini, L., Cassisi, G., & Sarzi-Puttini, P. (2014). Physiopathology of pain in rheumatology. *Reumatismo*, *66*(1), 4-13.

Cazzola, M., Sarzi-Puttini, P., Stisi, S., Di Franco, M., Bazzichi, L., Carignola, R., ... & Atzeni, F. (2008). Fibromyalgia syndrome: definition and diagnostic aspects. *Reumatismo*, *60*(s1), 3-14.

Choy, E. H. (2015). The role of sleep in pain and fibromyalgia. *Nature Reviews Rheumatology*, *11*(9), 513-520.

Clauw, D. J. (2001). Elusive syndromes: Treating the biologic basis of fibromyalgia and related syndromes. *Cleveland Clinic Journal of Medicine*, *68*(10), 830, 832–834.

Conversano, C., & Marchi, L. (2018). *Vivere con la fibromialgia: strategie psicologiche per affrontare il dolore cronico*. Edizioni Centro Studi Erickson.

Cooper, T. E., Derry, S., Wiffen, P. J., & Moore, R. A. (2017). Gabapentin for fibromyalgia pain in adults. *Cochrane Database of Systematic Reviews*, *1*.

Crofford, L. J. (2002). The hypothalamic–pituitary–adrenal axis in the pathogenesis of rheumatic diseases. *Endocrinology and Metabolism Clinics*, *31*(1), 1–13.

Crombez, G., Vlaeyen, J. W., Heuts, P. H., & Lysens, R. (1999). Pain-related fear is more disabling than pain itself: Evidence on the role of pain-related fear in chronic back pain disability. *Pain*, *80*(1–2), 329–339.

Del Rosso, A., & MADDALI BONGI, S. (2015). La fibromialgia. La malattia. In *La riabilitazione multidisciplinare del malato reumatico* (pp. 320–330). Maddali e Bruni.

Derry, S., Wiffen, P. J., Haeuser, W., Mücke, M., Tölle, T. R., Bell, R. F., & Moore, R. A. (2017). Oral nonsteroidal anti-inflammatory drugs for fibromyalgia in adults. *Cochrane Database of Systematic Reviews*, *3*.

Di Carlo, M., Cesaroni, P., & Salaffi, F. (2021). Neuropathic pain features suggestive of small fibre neuropathy in fibromyalgia syndrome: A clinical and ultrasonographic study on female patients. *Clin Exp Rheumatol*, *39*(Suppl 130), 102–107.

Dickenson, A. H. (1990). A cure for wind up: NMDA receptor antagonists as potential analgesics. *Trends in Pharmacological Sciences*, *11*(8), 307–309.

Dreyer, L., Kendall, S., Danneskiold-Samsøe, B., Bartels, E. M., & Bliddal, H. (2010). Mortality in a cohort of Danish patients with fibromyalgia: Increased frequency of suicide. *Arthritis & Rheumatism*, *62*(10), 3101–3108.

Dubner, R., & Hargreaves, K. M. (1989). The neurobiology of pain and its modulation. *The Clinical journal of pain*, *5*(2), S1-6.

Ferraccioli, G., Cavalieri, F., Salaffi, F., Fontana, S., Scita, F., Nolli, M., & Maestri, D. (1990). Neuroendocrinologic findings in primary fibromyalgia (soft tissue chronic pain syndrome) and in other chronic rheumatic conditions (rheumatoid arthritis, low back pain). *The Journal of rheumatology*, *17*(7), 869–873.

Fitzcharles, M.-A., Da Costa, D., & Pöyhiä, R. (2003). A study of standard care in fibromyalgia syndrome: A favorable outcome. *The Journal of rheumatology*, *30*(1), 154–159.

Fitzcharles, M.-A., Ste-Marie, P. A., Goldenberg, D. L., Pereira, J. X., Abbey, S., Choinière, M., Ko, G., Moulin, D. E., Panopalis, P., & Proulx, J. (2013). Canadian Pain Society and Canadian Rheumatology Association recommendations for rational care of persons with fibromyalgia. A summary report. *The Journal of rheumatology*, *40*(8), 1388–1393.

Friesen, L. N., Hadjistavropoulos, H. D., Schneider, L. H., Alberts, N. M., Titov, N., & Dear, B. F. (2017). Examination of an internet-delivered cognitive behavioural pain management course for adults with fibromyalgia: A randomized controlled trial. *Pain*, *158*(4), 593–604.

Gabuzda, D., & Wang, J. (1999). Chemokine receptors and virus entry in the central nervous system. *Journal of neurovirology*, *5*(6), 643–658.

Garrison, R. L., & Breeding, P. C. (2003). A metabolic basis for fibromyalgia and its related disorders: The possible role of resistance to thyroid hormone. *Medical hypotheses*, *61*(2), 182–189.

Garritano, F. (2023). *La fibromialgia è una sfida: tu puoi vincerla: Spiegazioni utili e consigli pratici per affrontare una sindrome reale e invalidante.* Edizioni LSWR.

Goldenberg, D. L., Clauw, D. J., Palmer, R. E., & Clair, A. G. (2016). Opioid use in fibromyalgia: A cautionary tale. *Mayo Clinic Proceedings*, *91*(5), 640–648.

Gowers, W. R. (1904). A lecture on lumbago: Its lessons and analogues: Delivered at the national hospital for the paralysed and epileptic. *British medical journal*, *1*(2246), 117.

Gracely, R. H., Petzke, F., Wolf, J. M., & Clauw, D. J. (2002). Functional magnetic resonance imaging evidence of augmented pain processing in fibromyalgia. *Arthritis & Rheumatism*, *46*(5), 1333–1343.

Greenfield, S., Fitzcharles, M.-A., & Esdaile, J. M. (1992). Reactive fibromyalgia syndrome. *Arthritis & Rheumatism: Official Journal of the American College of Rheumatology*, *35*(6), 678–681.

Griep, E. N., Boersma, J. W., & De Kloet, E. R. (1993). Altered reactivity of the hypothalamic-pituitary-adrenal axis in the primary fibromyalgia syndrome. *The Journal of rheumatology*, *20*(3), 469–474.

Hassett, A. L., Cone, J. D., Patella, S. J., & Sigal, L. H. (2000). The role of catastrophizing in the pain and depression of women with fibromyalgia syndrome. *Arthritis & Rheumatism: Official Journal of the American College of Rheumatology, 43*(11), 2493–2500.

Kosek, E., & Hansson, P. (1997). Modulatory influence on somatosensory perception from vibration and heterotopic noxious conditioning stimulation (HNCS) in fibromyalgia patients and healthy subjects. *Pain, 70*(1), 41–51.

Lauche, R., Cramer, H., Häuser, W., Dobos, G., & Langhorst, J. (2015). A systematic overview of reviews for complementary and alternative therapies in the treatment of the fibromyalgia syndrome. *Evidence-Based Complementary and Alternative Medicine, 2015*.

Lee, J., Protsenko, E., Lazaridou, A., Franceschelli, O., Ellingsen, D. M., Mawla, I., ... & Napadow, V. (2018). Encoding of self-referential pain catastrophizing in the posterior cingulate cortex in fibromyalgia. *Arthritis & rheumatology, 70*(8), 1308-1318.

Leskowitz, E. (2008). Energy-based therapies for chronic pain. *Integrative Pain Medicine: The science and practice of complementary and alternative medicine in pain management*, 225-241.

Li, J., Simone, D. A., & Larson, A. A. (1999). Windup leads to characteristics of central sensitization. *Pain, 79*(1), 75–82.

Macfarlane, G. J., Kronisch, C., Dean, L. E., Atzeni, F., Häuser, W., Fluß, E., Choy, E., Kosek, E., Amris, K., & Branco, J. (2017). EULAR revised recommendations for the management of fibromyalgia. *Annals of the rheumatic diseases, 76*(2), 318–328.

McKernan, L. C., Lenert, M. C., Crofford, L. J., & Walsh, C. G. (2019). Outpatient engagement and predicted risk of suicide attempts in fibromyalgia. *Arthritis care & research, 71*(9), 1255–1263.

Mease, P. (2005). Fibromyalgia syndrome: Review of clinical presentation, pathogenesis, outcome measures, and treatment. *The Journal of Rheumatology Supplement, 75*, 6–21.

Mendell, L. M., & Wall, P. D. (1965). Responses of single dorsal cord cells to peripheral cutaneous unmyelinated fibres. *Nature, 206*(4979), 97–99.

Moore, A., Wiffen, P., & Kalso, E. (2014). Antiepileptic drugs for neuropathic pain and fibromyalgia. *Jama*, *312*(2), 182–183.

Mundal, I., Gråwe, R. W., Bjørngaard, J. H., Linaker, O. M., & Fors, E. A. (2014). Psychosocial factors and risk of chronic widespread pain: An 11-year follow-up study—The HUNT study. *PAIN®*, *155*(8), 1555–1561.

Murakami, M., Osada, K., Ichibayashi, H., Mizuno, H., Ochiai, T., Ishida, M., Alev, L., & Nishioka, K. (2017). An open-label, long-term, phase III extension trial of duloxetine in Japanese patients with fibromyalgia. *Modern rheumatology*, *27*(4), 688–695.

O'Malley, P. G., Balden, E., Tomkins, G., Santoro, J., Kroenke, K., & Jackson, J. L. (2000). Treatment of fibromyalgia with antidepressants: A meta-analysis. *Journal of general internal medicine*, *15*, 659–666.

Perrot, S. (2019). Fibromyalgia: A misconnection in a multiconnected world? *European Journal of Pain*, *23*(5), 866–873.

Qaseem, A., Kansagara, D., Forciea, M. A., Cooke, M., Denberg, T. D., & Physicians*, C. G. C. of the A. C. of. (2016). Management of chronic insomnia disorder in adults: A clinical practice guideline from the American College of Physicians. *Annals of internal medicine*, *165*(2), 125–133.

Rahman, A., Underwood, M., & Carnes, D. (2014). Fibromyalgia. *Bmj*, 348.

Reisine, S., Fifield, J., Walsh, S., & Forrest, D. D. (2008). Employment and health status changes among women with fibromyalgia: A five-year study. *Arthritis Care & Research*, *59*(12), 1735–1741.

Ressler, K. J., & Nemeroff, C. B. (2000). Role of serotonergic and noradrenergic systems in the pathophysiology of depression and anxiety disorders. *Depression and anxiety*, *12*(S1), 2–19.

Rivera, J., De Diego, A., Trinchet, M., & Garcia Monforte, A. (1997). Fibromyalgia-associated hepatitis C virus infection. *British journal of rheumatology*, *36*(9), 981–985.

Roizenblatt, S., Moldofsky, H., Benedito-Silva, A. A., & Tufik, S. (2001). Alpha Sleep Characteristics in Fibromyalgia. *ARTHRITIS & RHEUMATISM*, *44*(1), 222–230.

Rosenbaum, S., Vancampfort, D., Steel, Z., Newby, J., Ward, P. B., & Stubbs, B. (2015). Physical activity in the treatment of post-traumatic stress disorder: A systematic review and meta-analysis. *Psychiatry research, 230*(2), 130–136.

Russell, I. J., & Raphael, K. G. (2008). Fibromyalgia syndrome: presentation, diagnosis, differential diagnosis, and vulnerability. *CNS spectrums, 13*(S5), 6-11.

Salaffi, F., & Sarzi-Puttini, P. (2012). Old and new criteria for the classification and diagnosis of fibromyalgia: comparison and evaluation. *Clin Exp Rheumatol, 30*(6 Suppl 74), 3-9.

Salaffi, F., Ciapetti, A., Puttini, P. S., Atzeni, F., Iannuccelli, C., Di Franco, M., ... & Bazzichi, L. (2012). Preliminary identification of key clinical domains for outcome evaluation in fibromyalgia using the Delphi method: the Italian experience. *Reumatismo, 64*(1), 27-34.

Salaffi, F., De Angelis, R., & Grassi, W. (2005). Prevalence of musculoskeletal conditions in an Italian population sample: results of a regional community-based study. I. The MAPPING study. *Clinical and experimental rheumatology, 23*(6), 819-828.

Salaffi, F., Giacobazzi, G., & Di Carlo, M. (2018). Chronic pain in inflammatory arthritis: mechanisms, metrology, and emerging targets—a focus on the JAK-STAT pathway. *Pain Research and Management, 2018.*

Salaffi, F., Mozzani, F., Draghessi, A., Atzeni, F., Catellani, R., Ciapetti, A., ... & Sarzi-Puttini, P. (2016). Identifying the symptom and functional domains in patients with fibromyalgia: results of a cross-sectional Internet-based survey in Italy. *Journal of Pain Research,* 279-286.

Salaffi, F., & Farah, S. (2019). *FIBROMIALGIA: EPIDEMIOLOGIA, INQUADRAMENTO CLINICO E CRITERI DIAGNOSTICI.* Rheumalab.

Sarzi-Puttini, P., Atzeni, F., Masala, I. F., Salaffi, F., Chapman, J., & Choy, E. (2018). Are the ACR 2010 diagnostic criteria for fibromyalgia better than the 1990 criteria?. *Autoimmunity reviews, 17*(1), 33-35.

Silva, A. R., Bernardo, A., Costa, J., Cardoso, A., Santos, P., de Mesquita, M. F., Vaz Patto, J., Moreira, P., Silva, M. L., & Padrão, P. (2019).

Dietary interventions in fibromyalgia: A systematic review. *Annals of medicine*, *51*(sup1), 2–14.

Staud, R., & Domingo, M. (2001). Evidence for abnormal pain processing in fibromyalgia syndrome. *Pain Medicine*, *2*(3), 208–215.

Staud, R., & Smitherman, M. L. (2002). Peripheral and central sensitization in fibromyalgia: Pathogenetic role. *Current pain and headache reports*, *6*, 259–266.

Staud, R., Cannon, R. C., Mauderli, A. P., Robinson, M. E., Price, D. D., & Vierck Jr, C. J. (2003). Temporal summation of pain from mechanical stimulation of muscle tissue in normal controls and subjects with fibromyalgia syndrome. *Pain*, *102*(1–2), 87–95.

Staud, R., Vierck, C. J., Cannon, R. L., Mauderli, A. P., & Price, D. D. (2001). Abnormal sensitization and temporal summation of second pain (wind-up) in patients with fibromyalgia syndrome. *Pain*, *91*(1–2), 165–175.

Stisi, S., Cazzola, M., Buskila, D., Spath, M., Giamberardino, M. A., Sarzi-Puttini, P., Arioli, G., Alciati, A., Leardini, G., & Gorla, R. (2008). Etiopathogenetic mechanisms of fibromyalgia syndrome. *Reumatismo-The Italian Journal of Rheumatology*, *60*(s1), 25–35.

Stubbs, B., Vancampfort, D., Rosenbaum, S., Firth, J., Cosco, T., Veronese, N., Salum, G. A., & Schuch, F. B. (2017). An examination of the anxiolytic effects of exercise for people with anxiety and stress-related disorders: A meta-analysis. *Psychiatry research*, *249*, 102–108.

Theadom, A., Cropley, M., Smith, H. E., Feigin, V. L., & McPherson, K. (2015). Mind and body therapy for fibromyalgia. *Cochrane Database of Systematic Reviews*, *4*.

Turk, D. C., & Okifuji, A. (2002). Psychological factors in chronic pain: Evolution and revolution. *Journal of consulting and clinical psychology*, *70*(3), 678.

Turk, D. C., Robinson, J. P., & Burwinkle, T. (2004). Prevalence of fear of pain and activity in patients with fibromyalgia syndrome. *The Journal of Pain*, *5*(9), 483–490.

Vlaeyen, J. W., de Jong, J., Geilen, M., Heuts, P. H., & van Breukelen, G. (2001). Graded exposure in vivo in the treatment of pain-related fear:

A replicated single-case experimental design in four patients with chronic low back pain. *Behaviour research and therapy*, *39*(2), 151–166.

Vlaeyen, J. W., Kole-Snijders, A. M., Rotteveel, A. M., Ruesink, R., & Heuts, P. H. (1995). The role of fear of movement/(re) injury in pain disability. *Journal of occupational rehabilitation*, *5*, 235–252.

Waddell, G., Newton, M., Henderson, I., Somerville, D., & Main, C. J. (1993). A Fear-Avoidance Beliefs Questionnaire (FABQ) and the role of fear-avoidance beliefs in chronic low back pain and disability. *Pain*, *52*(2), 157–168.

Walitt, B., Fitzcharles, M.-A., Hassett, A. L., Katz, R. S., Häuser, W., & Wolfe, F. (2011). The longitudinal outcome of fibromyalgia: A study of 1555 patients. *The Journal of rheumatology*, *38*(10), 2238–2246.

Watkins, L. R., & Maier, S. F. (2005). Immune regulation of central nervous system functions: From sickness responses to pathological pain. *Journal of internal medicine*, *257*(2), 139–155.

Watkins, L. R., Milligan, E. D., & Maier, S. F. (2001). Spinal cord glia: New players in pain. *Pain*, *93*(3), 201–205.

Wolfe, F. (2019). Letter to the editor,"Fibromyalgia Criteria". *The Journal of Pain*, *20*(6), 739-740.

Wolfe, F., Anderson, J., Harkness, D., Bennett, R. M., Caro, X. J., Goldenberg, D. L., Russell, I. J., & Yunus, M. B. (1997). Health status and disease severity in fibromyalgia. Results of a six-center longitudinal study. *Arthritis & Rheumatism: Official Journal of the American College of Rheumatology*, *40*(9), 1571–1579.

Wolfe, F., Clauw, D. J., Fitzcharles, M. A., Goldenberg, D. L., Häuser, W., Katz, R. S., ... & Winfield, J. B. (2011). Fibromyalgia criteria and severity scales for clinical and epidemiological studies: a modification of the ACR Preliminary Diagnostic Criteria for Fibromyalgia. *The Journal of rheumatology*, *38*(6), 1113-1122.

Wolfe, F., Clauw, D. J., Fitzcharles, M. A., Goldenberg, D. L., Katz, R. S., Mease, P., ... & Yunus, M. B. (2010). The American College of Rheumatology preliminary diagnostic criteria for fibromyalgia and measurement of symptom severity. *Arthritis care & research*, *62*(5), 600-610.

Wolfe, F., Smythe, H. A., Yunus, M. B., Bennett, R. M., Bombardier, C., Goldenberg, D. L., Tugwell, P., Campbell, S. M., Abeles, M., & Clark, P. (1990). The American College of Rheumatology 1990 criteria for the classification of fibromyalgia. *Arthritis & Rheumatism: Official Journal of the American College of Rheumatology*, *33*(2), 160–172.

Wolfe, F., Walitt, B. T., Katz, R. S., & Häuser, W. (2014). Social security work disability and its predictors in patients with fibromyalgia. *Arthritis care & research*, *66*(9), 1354–1363.

Younger, J., Noor, N., McCue, R., & Mackey, S. (2013). Low-dose naltrexone for the treatment of fibromyalgia: Findings of a small, randomized, double-blind, placebo-controlled, counterbalanced, crossover trial assessing daily pain levels. *Arthritis & Rheumatism*, *65*(2), 529–538.

Yunus, M. B. (1992). Towards a model of pathophysiology of fibromyalgia: Aberrant central pain mechanisms with peripheral modulation. *Journal of Rheumatology*, *19*(6), 846–850.

Chapter 2
THE BENEFITS OF ADAPTED PHYSICAL ACTIVITY TO INDIVIDUALS WITH FIBROMYALGIA

by G. Greco, V. Pugliese, F. Festa, F. Fischetti

2.1 The prescription of physical exercise as a non-pharmacological treatment

Physical exercise is defined as "a planned, structured and repeated physical activity aimed at improving and maintaining physical efficiency" (Caspersen et al., 1985). The goals of exercise in rheumatic diseases are to improve joint motility, muscle strength, and physical fitness. In the management of rheumatic diseases, both inflammatory and degenerative, exercise, in recent years, has replaced the immobilization and rest that were prescribed in the past, both in bed and through the use of braces and casts, which resulted in reduction of joint motility, to the point of inducing the development of ankylosis and a decrease in muscle strength, bone mineral density and cardiorespiratory function (Partridge & Duthie, 1963).

Fibromyalgia syndrome is one of the most widespread rheumatic diseases, with a clear prevalence in females. Chronic widespread musculoskeletal pain and asthenia are the fundamental symptoms, which, together with many others (sleep disorders, stiffness, depression, etc.), significantly reduce patients' quality of life. Therapy is difficult and no drug is truly effective, therefore treatment must be multidisciplinary. Personalized physical exercise is among the most important treatments, capable of interrupting the vicious pain-inactivity-pain cycle, reducing fatigue, and improving physical fitness and mood, often significantly compromised in fibromyalgia patients (Bongi & Del Rosso, 2010).

The American Pain Society (2005) and the Association of the Scientific Medical Societies in Germany (2008) assign a high level of recommendation to aerobic physical exercise during fibromyalgia syndrome, as part of a multidisciplinary treatment (Häuser et al., 2008). The 2007 Cochrane Review, comparing aerobic exercises (such as "stepping" and walking), muscle strengthening exercises (weightlifting or use of resistance equipment) and muscle lengthening exercises, concludes that there is strong evidence that Controlled aerobic training has beneficial effects on physical capacity and symptoms of fibromyalgia (FM). On the contrary, no conclusion is possible on the prescription of other types of exercise in fibromyalgia patients (Busch et al., 2007). Furthermore, to prevent physical activity from causing worsening of symptoms, in particular pain, reported in various studies, the Authors recommend increasing the intensity of training very slowly, checking the patient frequently, and, in case of an adverse event, reducing the intensity of the exercises until it disappears.

In 2008, the Ottawa Panel, based on scientific evidence, published recommendations regarding the performance of aerobic exercises and also muscle strengthening exercises for fibromyalgia patients (Brosseau, 2008). Certainly, in the evaluation of the various rheumatological rehabilitation studies, a limit is represented by the individualization of the exercises, which does not allow us to know exactly the type of movements performed and, therefore, makes it difficult to compare the results between the various methods used. Water exercises have demonstrated considerable effectiveness, although short-lived, in reducing pain and the number of tender points and in improving health in a recent review conducted on 10 articles selected from the 1900 published from 1990 to 2006 (McVeigh, 2008).

However, clinical experience suggests that the optimal rehabilitation approach for FM may be represented by gentle gymnastics, which involve a global body-mind involvement, particularly suitable for the complex psychological-functional alterations of the fibromyalgia patient. At the moment, there is only some scientific evidence, which shows, however, promising results of some methods, such as Qi Gong (Haak & Scott, 2008) and Tai Chi (Taggart et al., 2003).

Movement approaches such as dance therapy, biodance or aquatic biodance have proven effective in rehabilitation programs for FM (Carbonell-Baeza et al., 2010).

Results relating to the physical symptoms of people suffering from FM differ depending on the therapy; a basic therapy, based on body awareness, can be defined as a therapy that focuses on the internal subjective experience of the body (Mehling et al., 2011), a holistic therapy aimed at awareness of how the body works, how it is used, of how he interacts with himself and others (Gard, 2005), promotes physical, mental and emotional well-being, showing a significant improvement in pain levels.

Furthermore, Liu et al. (2012) studied how Qi Gong improves general pain and functional limitations, comparing two Qi Gong modalities that both led to improvements in general pain.

Regarding the effect on psychological aspects, body awareness therapies that demonstrate the best effects are Qi Gong, Tai Chi, strengthening programs, and yoga (Bravo et al., 2019).

Recent scientific literature indicates several biological mechanisms that may explain the therapeutic effects of exercise in patients with FM. The effects of exercise are not limited to a single physiological system and can affect the entire individual. Regular physical exercise may have the ability to influence the nociceptive, neuroendocrine, and autonomic systems, along with cognitive abilities and mood disorders in individuals with FM. As regards the nociceptive system, the hypothesis of an effect of exercise on the descending modulation of pain has its own significance; Cardiovascular fitness training three times a week for 20 weeks increases the level of serotonin and its metabolite 5-hydroxyindole acetic acid (5-HIAA), suggesting stimulation of descending pain modulation (Valim et al., 2013). Furthermore, the authors observed that physically more active FM subjects were better able to modulate repeated painful thermal stimuli than minimally active FM subjects (McLoughlin et al., 2015).

The hypothesis of the effect of physical exercise on the hypothalamic-pituitary-adrenal axis was formulated based on the study by Genc et al. (2015) who proposed 6 weeks of aerobic exercises in 50 fibromyalgia subjects. This led to reduction in pain, morning stiffness and a significant increase in growth hormone along with a significant reduction in serum cortisol levels (Genc et al., 2015).

A systematic review demonstrated that moderate to vigorous aerobic exercise performed twice a week was effective in reducing autonomic nervous system dysfunction and increasing heart rate variability. Furthermore, strength training reduced symptoms of anxiety and depression while improving muscle strength in patients with FM (Andrade et al., 2019).

2.2 The effects of adapted physical activity on the pain neuromodulation process

As already highlighted several times, the main symptom of FM is widespread pain, mainly in the muscles and joints, which compromises the functional abilities of the subjects. The symptoms most frequently associated with pain and described by patients with FM are chronic fatigue, sleep disorders, cognitive disorders, and emotional disorders (Cánovas et al., 2009) . This symptomatology then leads to a serious deterioration in the quality of life, sometimes with physical disabilities leading to social isolation and difficulty maintaining employment (recurrent sickness absence). There is currently no etiological treatment for FM, however, all pain associations and best practice guidelines strongly support the practice of physical activity to improve the symptoms of subjects with FM (Le Fur Bonnabesse et al., 2019) .

Corticotropic axis malfunction has often been described in FM, which also signals stress axis dysfunction; in fact, the mechanisms that determine dysfunctional pain, in FM and beyond, are mostly central and linked precisely to the dysfunction of this axis (autonomic nervous system and adeno-corticotropic axis) (Woda et al., 2013) . The main indicator of stress axis dysfunction is often determined by an imbalance between the sympathetic and parasympathetic responses. At rest, patients with FM show an increase in the response associated with the sympathetic component of the nervous system, and at the same time there is a decrease in parasympathetic tone (da Cunha Ribeiro et al., 2011) , this situation is defined as neurovegetative dystonia (Martinez-Lavin, 2004) . However, the form this dysfunction takes differs (Tak et al., 2011) , but, whatever their form, all these dysfunctions compromise the body's adaptation to daily stressful stimuli.

Studies have therefore shown that this stress axis deficit (vegetative neurodystonia and dysfunctional corticotropic axis) is concomitant with FM (Clauw & Ablin, 2009) and is associated with impaired pain control (Woda et al., 2009) .

The pain control system and the stress axis have close anatomical and functional links. The nociceptive, autonomic, and corticotropic systems all interact with the central nervous system and the central neuromediators involved in the regulation of the stress axis are mostly common to those of pain neuromodulation (endogenous opioids, norepinephrine, serotonin, etc.) (Le Fur Bonnabesse et al., 2019).

To better understand how this dysfunction works and therefore identify the pain neuromodulation process underlying FM, we can consider an example, therefore referring to an overtrained elite athlete. The physical and psychological strain of training is known to induce stress, and elite athletes may exhibit overtraining syndrome when adaptive limits of the stress axis are reached. This stress-induced phenomenon corresponds to an imbalance between the amount of training and recovery. Overtrained athletes present a deconditioning syndrome close to the symptoms of FM (chronic pain, sleep disorders, autonomic dystonia, intense fatigue, etc.) (Kajaia et al., 2017).

However, most studies have shown that adequate and adapted physical activity is more effective on FM symptoms than pharmacological treatments (Fontenele & Felix, 2012). Literature reviews and meta-analyses strongly support the benefits of physical training in patients with FM (decreased pain and depression and improved general and physical health) (Busch et al., 2011). The practice of aerobic exercise in patients with FM is strongly recommended by the American Pain Society (American Pain Society, 2005), the Association of Medical-Scientific Societies in Germany (Häuser et al., 2008), the Canadian Rheumatology Association (Fitzcharles et al., 2013) and by the European League

Against Rheumatism (Macfarlane et al., 2017). These recommendations occur above all because constant physical activity is associated with cardiovascular benefits, but not only that, it acts above all at the level of the autonomic nervous system and therefore on the process of neuromodulation of pain. One of the benefits associated with physical activity occurs in the increase in parasympathetic tone associated with a decrease in the sympathetic response (Martins -Pinge, 2011), elements which we have seen to be altered in the process of neuromodulation of pain in FM and which with physical activity can be rebalanced. The mechanisms and structures involved in the activation and regulation of the autonomic nervous system interact with the central nervous system, and the central relationships between the autonomic nervous system and the motor cortex, limbic system, hypothalamus, pituitary gland, and basal ganglia determine the release of analgesic neurotransmitters such as norepinephrine, serotonin and endogenous opioids (Santos & Galdino, 2018). This release of neurotransmitters due to exercise leads to an increase in endogenous inhibition and therefore a decrease in widespread pain in FM (Brito et al., 2017). Therefore the plasticity of the central nervous system, induced by physical training, will certainly regulate cardiovascular adaptations, a concept that appears to be better known, but at the same time it will also regulate the endogenous mechanisms of pain control (Naugle et al., 2014). Therefore, strategies to rebalance the autonomic system, among which physical activity can be considered the most important, are the most promising therapies for FM (de Abreu et al., 2009).

2.3 The effects of different types of activity on physical abilities and functional status

The basic principle, on which the relationship between physical activity and FM is based, is certainly determined by what has been the demonstration of the significant improvement with respect to pain and functional activity in individuals with FM, which physical exercise determines (Macfarlane et al., 2017). Individuals with FM can perform different types of exercise (Häuser et al., 2010). Regular exercise is an important factor in counteracting age-related loss of muscle mass, bone mass and functional independence for the general population; therefore, individuals with FM can improve their overall health and moderate the risks associated with other chronic conditions by following an exercise program. Most research studies involve the use of different training protocols, which can mainly be identified as activities that individually refer to some specific parameters, including aerobic resistance, flexibility and strength above all (Busch et al., 2009). Individuals with FM are often characterized by poor cardiovascular fitness (Turk, 2020), muscular strength, and muscular endurance (Bennett & Walczyk, 1998).

Regarding aerobic endurance, according to the American College of Sports Medicine (ACSM) guidelines for exercise testing and prescription, aerobic exercise (also called cardiorespiratory or resistance exercise) represents a wide range of physical activities such as walking, jogging, cycling, and dancing performed at sub-maximal intensities that can be sustained for minutes to hours, depending on the fitness level of the individual and the intensity of the exercise. Aerobic training represents organized regimes of physical activity that are repeated over time (ACSM, 2013). Aerobic exercise is the most easily accessible and most commonly recognized form of exercise, making it a reasonable recommendation and treatment strategy (Eyler et al., 2003) . Moderate and vigorous programs of aerobic training and leisure-time physical activity have been shown to improve physical fitness, and reduce the risk of mortality and morbidity from all causes and cardiovascular disease (Garber et al., 2011) . In its position paper, the ACSM recommends that for aerobic exercise, most adults should engage in moderate-intensity cardiorespiratory exercise using large muscle groups and rhythmic activities for 30 minutes or more per day for five or more days at a time. week for a total of 150 minutes or more; or vigorous-intensity cardiorespiratory exercise training for 20 minutes or more per day for three or more days per week for a total of 75 minutes or more per week; or a combination of moderate- and vigorous-intensity exercise performed to achieve a total energy expenditure of between 500 and 1000 metabolic equivalents (METs) per week. Aerobic exercise alters neurotransmitters, neuromodulators, brain chemistry, and hypothalamic-pituitary function (Klaperski et al., 2014). These elements are involved in brain function and their improvement through exercise can lead to improved feelings of energy, improved mood, and a reduction in stress, anxiety, and depression (Moylan et al., 2013). With aerobic exercise, the hypothalamus releases increased levels of neurotransmitters including endorphins (Lopresti et al., 2013).

This increase in endorphin release results in a decrease in pain sensation and an improvement in mood states and sleep quality (Scheef et al., 2012).

Exercise can contribute to pain reduction by improving the physiological response to muscle microtrauma through increased resilience, repair, and subsequent adaptation (McLoughlin et al., 2011). Aerobic exercise also leads to a reduction in inflammation and oxidative stress in the body, which results in reduced anxiety and stress responses (Moylan et al., 2013). Aerobic exercise has been found to improve feelings of energy and fatigue in various medical conditions, including FM (Puetz et al., 2006). Since high levels of fatigue have been associated with low levels of physical activity and impaired physical capacity in FM (Ericsson et al., 2013), the improvement of physical capacity, achieved through aerobic activity, in patients with FM may lead to reducing fatigue and consequently improving the subject's functional capabilities. Overall, aerobic exercise can help improve physiology, which can attenuate alterations associated with FM (Ericsson et al., 2016).

About flexibility exercise training, these are protocols that focus on improving or maintaining the range of motion of muscles and joint structures by holding or lengthening the body in specific positions (ACSM, 2013). The joint range of motion is an important physical characteristic that influences the ability to perform activities of daily living (Mulholland & Wyss, 2001). Muscle stretching exercises increase the length of the muscle (or muscle group) beyond what would normally be used in normal activity. Low levels of flexibility have been associated with postural problems, pain, injury, decreased local vascularity, and increased neuromuscular tension (dos Santos Coelho, 2008). Indeed, flexibility training programs have been used to improve a person's well-being and as a tool for symptom management in several clinical populations such as those with major depressive disorders (Ambrose & Golightly, 2015).

The primary goal of flexibility training is usually to improve or maintain range of motion in major muscle-tendon groups by individualized goals (Garber et al., 2011). Flexibility training improves postural stability and balance (Costa et al., 2009), and improves physical function, range of motion and muscle strength (Jones et al., 2006). In this sense, these types of training also reduce FM symptoms such as pain (Valencia et al., 2009), muscle stiffness, fatigue, and psychological factors associated with anxiety and depression) (Lanuez et al., 2011). Good flexibility training would also improve proprioception, a quality that is also useful for carrying out daily life activities (Soriano-Maldonado et al., 2016). Flexibility training can therefore be useful for both improving fitness and controlling symptoms. Because stiffness and reduced range of motion have been shown to reduce health-related quality of life in individuals with FM, flexibility training may help reduce these physical difficulties, thereby improving the functional status of the subjects (Valencia et al., 2009).

As we have seen, the activity protocols are different and contribute in different ways to improving the lives of those affected by FM. However, it has been suggested that there are no physical activity parameters that are universal, parameters such as the dose of physical exercise, the intensity of exercise, and the type of exercise must be adapted to the needs of the individual (Eijsvogels & Thompson, 2015). In research on the effectiveness of exercise, the type of exercise and dose are usually standardized. This means that the type of physical activity performed is usually not determined by the patient but by the clinical research team, and therefore may not actually be appropriate for individuals (Busch et al., 2009).

A fundamental role in general appears to be played by multidisciplinary treatments (of which physical activity is part); these have proven effective in reducing the impact and level of pain associated with FM (Castel et al., 2013), but above all, they have been identified as successfully improving the "functional status" (Marcus et al., 2014) which is defined as "an individual's ability to carry out normal daily activities necessary to meet basic needs, fulfill habitual roles, and maintain health and wellbeing (Wilson & Cleary, 1995)".

2.4 The effectiveness of body awareness therapies associated with fibromyalgia

A fundamental element to consider in the quality of life and the effectiveness of daily activities is certainly the so-called "body schema". This concept is fundamental for everyone's life, but in particular for those affected by FM, as the sedentary lifestyle associated with this pathology very often leads to a distortion of vision and consideration of one's body image. In this sense, therefore, some types of physical activity are extremely effective for these patients we are talking about what is defined as body awareness therapy (Bravo Navarro et al., 2019). Movement awareness is a term that can be described as sensitivity to different nuances of movement, becoming aware of how movements are performed and experienced in relation to space, time, and energy, as well as identifying movement reactions in relation to conditions internal, environmental, and relational (Skjaerven et al., 2019).

Examples of movement awareness therapies within physical therapy include basic "body awareness" (BA) therapy. BA therapies refer to a group of interventions that share a common perspective that focuses on the internal subjective experience of the body (Mehling et al., 2011).

Therefore, BA therapies can be defined as body-oriented therapeutic approaches, which use a holistic perspective, directed at awareness of how the body is used, in terms of bodily function, behavior, and interaction with self and others (Gard, 2005). This group of interventions promotes physical, mental and emotional well-being.

Although the classification of BA therapies remains unclear as there are other approaches and traditions in the field, Eastern approaches such as Tai Chi, Qi Gong, and yoga can be considered among them. These activities represent meditative movement traditions that are determined by forms of movement and body positioning, achieved by focusing on breathing and a clear and calm state of mind with the aim of creating deep states of relaxation (Langhorst et al., 2013).

BA therapies have shown positive results in several pathologies such as cancer (Zeng et al., 2014) in terms of physical, psychological, and immune function (Morgan et al., 2014), quality of life, and bone density (Jahnke et al., 2010). European movement approaches such as dance therapy such as biodance and aquatic biodance have demonstrated effectiveness in rehabilitation programs for FM (Carbonell-Baeza et al., 2010). The positive effects and effectiveness of these programs on FM have been identified at various levels, starting from physical symptoms up to good results from a physiological point of view. Outcomes related to the physical symptoms of people with FM differ depending on the therapy. Basic BA therapy (Bravo et al., 2019) showed significant improvement in pain levels. In terms of affective self-awareness (ASA) (Hsu et al., 2010), approximately half of the participants treated in the different studies showed a reduction in pain of at least 30% and the results were maintained even at the six-year follow-up. months. One study in particular, which combined Qi Gong and BA therapy achieved an improvement in movement harmony, however this approach should be further analyzed due to the small number of subjects and high dropout rate (Mannerkorpi & Arndorw, 2004). Furthermore, Qi Gong, yoga, and physical activity associated with a good lifestyle have been shown to improve all symptoms such as general pain, quality of movement, functional limitations, and quality of life. Dance therapy, biodance, and aquatic biodance in various studies also generally led to an improvement in pain (Bravo Navarro et al., 2019).

BA therapies that show effects on psychological outcomes are mindfulness-based cognitive therapy, affective self-awareness (ASA), Qi Gong, Tai Chi, and yoga. Cognitive and mindfulness meditation plus Qi Gong improve symptoms of depression (Astin et al., 2003).

While aquatic biodance has proven useful in achieving an improvement in anxiety symptoms (López-Rodríguez et al., 2012). Yoga, on the other hand, has been shown to reduce anxiety by

42.2%, depression by 41.5%, and emotional distress by 30.1% (Carson et al., 2010).

Finally, the effectiveness also occurred at a physiological level. People diagnosed with FM also suffer from physiological symptoms such as sleep disturbances and fatigue. ASA, in several studies, has been shown to result in less post-treatment fatigue (Bravo Navarro et al., 2019). Tai Chi instead determines an improvement in the quality of sleep (Jones et al., 2012). Qi Gong shows a 37.3% decrease in sleep disturbances and a 24.8% reduction in fatigue (Liu et al., 2012). Furthermore, yoga has shown a beneficial reduction in fatigue by 29.9% (Carson et al., 2010), while dance has also shown significant improvements in sleep quality (Astin et al., 2003).

References

Ambrose, K. R., & Golightly, Y. M. (2015). Physical exercise as non-pharmacological treatment of chronic pain: Why and when. *Best practice & research Clinical rheumatology*, *29*(1), 120–130.

Andrade, A., Steffens, R. D. A. K., Sieczkowska, S. M., Tartaruga, L. A. P., & Vilarino, G. T. (2019). A systematic review of the effects of strength training in patients with fibromyalgia: clinical outcomes and design considerations. *Advances in rheumatology, 58*.

Bennett, R. M., & Walczyk, J. (1998). A randomized, double-blind, placebo-controlled study of growth hormone in the treatment of fibromyalgia. *The American journal of medicine*, *104*(3), 227–231.

Bongi, S. M., & Del Rosso, A. (2010). How to prescribe physical exercise in rheumatology. *Reumatismo*, *62*(1), 4-11.

Bravo, C., Skjaerven, L. H., Sein-Echaluce, L. G., & Catalan-Matamoros, D. (2019). Effectiveness of movement and body awareness therapies in patients with fibromyalgia: a systematic review and meta-analysis. *Eur J Phys Rehabil Med, 55*(5), 646-657.

Brito, R. G., Rasmussen, L. A., & Sluka, K. A. (2017). Regular physical activity prevents development of chronic muscle pain through modulation of supraspinal opioid and serotonergic mechanisms. *Pain reports*, *2*(5).

Brosseau, L., Wells, G. A., Tugwell, P., Egan, M., Wilson, K. G., Dubouloz, C. J., ... & Veilleux, L. (2008). Ottawa Panel evidence-based clinical practice guidelines for aerobic fitness exercises in the management of fibromyalgia: part 1. *Physical therapy*, *88*(7), 857-871.

Busch, A. J., Barber, K. A., Overend, T. J., Peloso, P. M. J., & Schachter, C. L. (2007). Exercise for treating fibromyalgia syndrome. *Cochrane database of systematic reviews*, (4).

Busch, A. J., Overend, T. J., & Schachter, C. L. (2009). Fibromyalgia treatment: The role of exercise and physical activity. *Int J Clin Rheumtol, 4*(3), 343–380.

Busch, A. J., Webber, S. C., Brachaniec, M., Bidonde, J., Bello-Haas, V. D., Danyliw, A. D., Overend, T. J., Richards, R. S., Sawant, A., &

Schachter, C. L. (2011). Exercise therapy for fibromyalgia. *Current pain and headache reports*, *15*, 358–367.

Cánovas, R., León, I., Roldán, M. D., Astur, R., & Cimadevilla, J. M. (2009). Virtual reality tasks disclose spatial memory alterations in fibromyalgia. *Rheumatology*, *48*(10), 1273–1278.

Carbonell-Baeza, A., Aparicio, V. A., Martins-Pereira, C. M., Gatto-Cardia, C. M., Ortega, F. B., Huertas, F. J., ... & Delgado-Fernandez, M. (2010). Efficacy of Biodanza for treating women with fibromyalgia. *The journal of alternative and complementary medicine*, *16*(11), 1191-1200.

Caspersen, C. J., Powell, K. E., & Christenson, G. M. (1985). Physical activity, exercise, and physical fitness: definitions and distinctions for health-related research. *Public health reports*, *100*(2), 126.

Castel, A., Fontova, R., Montull, S., Periñán, R., Poveda, M. J., Miralles, I., Cascón-Pereira, R., Hernández, P., Aragonés, N., & Salvat, I. (2013). Efficacy of a multidisciplinary fibromyalgia treatment adapted for women with low educational levels: A randomized controlled trial. *Arthritis care & research*, *65*(3), 421–431.

Clauw, D. J., & Ablin, J. N. (2009). The relationship between "stress" and pain: Lessons learned from fibromyalgia and related conditions. *Current topics in pain: 12th world congress on pain*, 245–271.

Costa, P. B., Graves, B. S., Whitehurst, M., & Jacobs, P. L. (2009). The acute effects of different durations of static stretching on dynamic balance performance. *The Journal of Strength & Conditioning Research*, *23*(1), 141–147.

da Cunha Ribeiro, R. P., Roschel, H., Artioli, G. G., Dassouki, T., Perandini, L. A., Calich, A. L., de Sá Pinto, A. L., Lima, F. R., Bonfá, E., & Gualano, B. (2011). Cardiac autonomic impairment and chronotropic incompetence in fibromyalgia. *Arthritis research & therapy*, *13*, 1–5.

de Abreu, S. B., Lenhard, A., Mehanna, A., de Souza, H. C. D., de Aguiar Correa, F. M., Hasser, E. M., & Martins-Pinge, M. C. (2009). Role of paraventricular nucleus in exercise training-induced autonomic modulation in conscious rats. *Autonomic Neuroscience*, *148*(1–2), 28–35.

dos Santos Coelho, L. F. (2008). The muscular flexibility training and the range of movement improvement: A critical literature review/O treino da flexibilidade muscular eo aumento da amplitude de movimento: Uma revisao critica da literatura. *Motricidade*, *4*(4), 59–71.

Eijsvogels, T. M., & Thompson, P. D. (2015). Exercise is medicine: At any dose? *Jama*, *314*(18), 1915–1916.

Ericsson, A., Bremell, T., & Mannerkorpi, K. (2013). Usefulness of multiple dimensions of fatigue in fibromyalgia. *Journal of Rehabilitation Medicine*, *45*(7), 685–693.

Ericsson, A., Palstam, A., Larsson, A., Löfgren, M., Bileviciute-Ljungar, I., Bjersing, J., Gerdle, B., Kosek, E., & Mannerkorpi, K. (2016). Resistance exercise improves physical fatigue in women with fibromyalgia: A randomized controlled trial. *Arthritis research & therapy*, *18*, 1–12.

Eyler, A. A., Brownson, R. C., Bacak, S. J., & Housemann, R. A. (2003). The epidemiology of walking for physical activity in the United States. *Medicine & Science in Sports & Exercise*, *35*(9), 1529–1536.

Fitzcharles, M.-A., Ste-Marie, P. A., Goldenberg, D. L., Pereira, J. X., Abbey, S., Choinière, M., Ko, G., Moulin, D. E., Panopalis, P., & Proulx, J. (2013). Canadian Pain Society and Canadian Rheumatology Association recommendations for rational care of persons with fibromyalgia. A summary report. *The Journal of rheumatology*, *40*(8), 1388–1393.

Fontenele, J. B., & Felix, F. H. C. (2012). Exercise for fibromyalgia: Evidence for an integrated modulation of autonomic and nociception neural regulation. *Rheumatology international*, *32*, 4075–4076.

Garber, C. E., Blissmer, B., Deschenes, M. R., Franklin, B. A., Lamonte, M. J., Lee, I.-M., Nieman, D. C., & Swain, D. P. (2011). American College of Sports Medicine position stand. Quantity and quality of exercise for developing and maintaining cardiorespiratory, musculoskeletal, and neuromotor fitness in apparently healthy adults: Guidance for prescribing exercise. *Medicine and science in sports and exercise*, *43*(7), 1334–1359.

Gard, G. (2005). Body awareness therapy for patients with fibromyalgia and chronic pain. *Disability and rehabilitation,* *27*(12), 725-728.

Genc, A., Tur, B. S., Aytur, Y. K., Oztuna, D., & Erdogan, M. F. (2015). Does aerobic exercise affect the hypothalamic-pituitary-adrenal hormonal response in patients with fibromyalgia syndrome?. *Journal of Physical Therapy Science, 27*(7), 2225-2231.

Haak, T., & Scott, B. (2008). The effect of Qigong on fibromyalgia (FMS): a controlled randomized study. *Disability and rehabilitation, 30*(8), 625-633.

Häuser, W., Arnold, B., Eich, W., Felde, E., Flügge, C., Henningsen, P., Herrmann, M., Köllner, V., Kühn, E., & Nutzinger, D. (2008). Management of fibromyalgia syndrome–an interdisciplinary evidence-based guideline. *GMS German Medical Science, 6*.

Häuser, W., Thieme, K., & Turk, D. C. (2010). Guidelines on the management of fibromyalgia syndrome–a systematic review. *European journal of pain, 14*(1), 5–10.

Jones, K. D., Adams, D., Winters-Stone, K., & Burckhardt, C. S. (2006). A comprehensive review of 46 exercise treatment studies in fibromyalgia (1988–2005). *Health and quality of life outcomes, 4*, 1–6.

Kajaia, T., Maskhulia, L., Chelidze, K., Akhalkatsi, V., & Kakhabrishvili, Z. (2017). The effects of non-functional overreaching and overtraining on autonomic nervous system function in highly trained Georgian athletes. *Georgian Medical Newa, 3*(264), 97–101.

Klaperski, S., von Dawans, B., Heinrichs, M., & Fuchs, R. (2014). Effects of a 12-week endurance training program on the physiological response to psychosocial stress in men: A randomized controlled trial. *Journal of behavioral medicine, 37*, 1118–1133.

Lanuez, F. V., Jacob-Filho, W., Lanuez, M. V., & Oliveira, A. C. B. de. (2011). Comparative study of the effects of two programs of physical exercises in flexibility and balance of healthy elderly individuals with and without major depression. *Einstein (São Paulo), 9*, 307–312.

Le Fur Bonnabesse, A., Cabon, M., L'Heveder, G., Kermarrec, A., Quinio, B., Woda, A., Marchand, S., Dubois, A., Giroux-Metges, M.-A., Rannou, F., Misery, L., & Bodéré, C. (2019). Impact of a specific training programme on the neuromodulation of pain in female patient with fibromyalgia (DouFiSport): A 24-month, controlled, randomised, double-blind protocol. *BMJ Open*, *9*(1), e023742. https://doi.org/10.1136/bmjopen-2018-023742

Liu, W., Zahner, L., Cornell, M., Le, T., Ratner, J., Wang, Y., ... & Barohn, R. (2012). Benefit of Qigong exercise in patients with fibromyalgia: a pilot study. *International Journal of Neuroscience*, *122*(11), 657-664.

Lopresti, A. L., Hood, S. D., & Drummond, P. D. (2013). A review of lifestyle factors that contribute to important pathways associated with major depression: Diet, sleep and exercise. *Journal of affective disorders*, *148*(1), 12–27.

Macfarlane, G. J., Kronisch, C., Dean, L. E., Atzeni, F., Häuser, W., Fluß, E., Choy, E., Kosek, E., Amris, K., & Branco, J. (2017). EULAR revised recommendations for the management of fibromyalgia. *Annals of the rheumatic diseases*, *76*(2), 318–328.

Marcus, D. A., Bernstein, C. D., Haq, A., & Breuer, P. (2014). Including a range of outcome targets offers a broader view of fibromyalgia treatment outcome: Results from a retrospective review of multidisciplinary treatment. *Musculoskeletal Care*, *12*(2), 74–81.

Martinez-Lavin, M. (2004). Fibromyalgia as a sympathetically maintained pain syndrome. *Current pain and headache reports*, *8*, 385–389.

Martins-Pinge, M. C. (2011). Cardiovascular and autonomic modulation by the central nervous system after aerobic exercise training. *Brazilian Journal of Medical and Biological Research*, *44*, 848–854.

McLoughlin, M. J., Stegner, A. J., & Cook, D. B. (2011). The relationship between physical activity and brain responses to pain in fibromyalgia. *The journal of pain*, *12*(6), 640–651.

McVeigh, J. G., McGaughey, H., Hall, M., & Kane, P. (2008). The effectiveness of hydrotherapy in the management of fibromyalgia syndrome: a systematic review. *Rheumatology international*, *29*, 119-130.

Mehling, W. E., Wrubel, J., Daubenmier, J. J., Price, C. J., Kerr, C. E., Silow, T., ... & Stewart, A. L. (2011). Body Awareness: a phenomenological inquiry into the common ground of mind-body therapies. *Philosophy, ethics, and humanities in medicine*, *6*(1), 1-12.

Moylan, S., Eyre, H. A., Maes, M., Baune, B. T., Jacka, F. N., & Berk, M. (2013). Exercising the worry away: How inflammation, oxidative and nitrogen stress mediates the beneficial effect of physical activity on anxiety disorder symptoms and behaviours. *Neuroscience & Biobehavioral Reviews*, *37*(4), 573–584.

Mulholland, S. J., & Wyss, U. P. (2001). Activities of daily living in non-Western cultures: Range of motion requirements for hip and knee joint implants. *International Journal of Rehabilitation Research*, *24*(3), 191–198.

Naugle, K. M., Naugle, K. E., Fillingim, R. B., Samuels, B., & Riley III, J. L. (2014). Intensity thresholds for aerobic exercise–induced hypoalgesia. *Medicine and science in sports and exercise*, *46*(4), 817.

Partridge, R. E. H., & Duthie, J. J. R. (1963). Controlled trial of the effect of complete immobilization of the joints in rheumatoid arthritis. *Annals of the rheumatic diseases*, *22*(2), 91.

Puetz, T. W., Beasman, K. M., & O'Connor, P. J. (2006). The effect of cardiac rehabilitation exercise programs on feelings of energy and fatigue: A meta-analysis of research from 1945 to 2005. *European Journal of Preventive Cardiology*, *13*(6), 886–893.

Santos, R. D. S., & Galdino, G. (2018). Endogenous systems involved in exercise-induced analgesia. *JPP*, *1*(01).

Scheef, L., Jankowski, J., Daamen, M., Weyer, G., Klingenberg, M., Renner, J., Mueckter, S., Schürmann, B., Musshoff, F., & Wagner, M. (2012). An fMRI study on the acute effects of exercise on pain processing in trained athletes. *PAIN®*, *153*(8), 1702–1714.

Soriano-Maldonado, A., Estévez-López, F., Segura-Jimenez, V., Aparicio, V. A., Alvarez-Gallardo, I. C., Herrador-Colmenero, M., Ruiz, J. R., Henriksen, M., Amris, K., & Delgado-Fernandez, M. (2016). Association of physical fitness with depression in women with fibromyalgia. *Pain Medicine*, *17*(8), 1542–1552.

Taggart, H. M., Arslanian, C. L., Bae, S., & Singh, K. (2003). Effects of T'ai Chi exercise on fibromyalgia symptoms and health-related quality of life. *Orthopaedic Nursing*, *22*(5), 353-360.

Tak, L. M., Cleare, A. J., Ormel, J., Manoharan, A., Kok, I. C., Wessely, S., & Rosmalen, J. G. (2011). Meta-analysis and meta-regression of hypothalamic-pituitary-adrenal axis activity in functional somatic disorders. *Biological psychology, 87*(2), 183–194.

Turk, D. C. (2020). Suffering and dysfunction in fibromyalgia syndrome. In *The Clinical Neurobiology of Fibromyalgia and Myofascial Pain* (pp. 85–96). CRC Press.

Valencia, M., Alonso, B., Alvarez, M. J., Barrientos, M. J., Ayán, C., & Sánchez, V. M. (2009). Effects of 2 physiotherapy programs on pain perception, muscular flexibility, and illness impact in women with fibromyalgia: A pilot study. *Journal of manipulative and physiological therapeutics, 32*(1), 84–92.

Valim, V., Natour, J., Xiao, Y., Pereira, A. F. A., da Cunha Lopes, B. B., Pollak, D. F., ... & Russell, I. J. (2013). Effects of physical exercise on serum levels of serotonin and its metabolite in fibromyalgia: a randomized pilot study. *Revista Brasileira De Reumatologia (English Edition), 53*(6), 538-541.

Woda, A., Dao, T., & Gremeau-Richard, C. (2009). Steroid dysregulation and stomatodynia (burning mouth syndrome). *Journal of orofacial pain, 23*(3).

Woda, A., L'heveder, G., Ouchchane, L., & Bodéré, C. (2013). Effect of experimental stress in 2 different pain conditions affecting the facial muscles. *The Journal of Pain, 14*(5), 455–466.

Chapter 3
PHYSICAL ACTIVITY AND PSYCHOPHYSICAL WELLBEING IN SUBJECTS WITH FIBROMYALGIA

by F. Fischetti, F. Festa, V. Pugliese, G. Greco

3.1 Physical activity and psychological wellbeing

The beneficial effects of physical activity in patients suffering from fibromyalgia (FM) do not only occur on a physical level, but they are also above all related to mental health. In addition to the core symptom of pain, patients with FM typically experience several additional symptoms, including sleep disturbances, fatigue, cognitive difficulties, depression, and anxiety (Jones et al., 2008). Physical activity in this sense can also help to modulate these aspects, improving the quality of life, not only in terms of daily activities but also of psychological well-being. The implementation of exercise as medicine has been recommended as an effective treatment for a broad spectrum of psychiatric illnesses (Pedersen & Saltin, 2015) and, as an evidence-based alternative to current recommendations, can simultaneously address comorbidity with several physical conditions frequently associated with mental health problems (World Health Organization, 2013). Indeed, evidence from many studies provides consistent support for physical activity interventions in reducing symptoms of depression (Cooney et al., 2013), anxiety (Stubbs et al., 2017), and stress disorder. post-traumatic stress (PTSD) (Rosenbaum et al., 2015), especially when compared with interventions that involve exclusively pharmacological treatment (Thomas et al., 2020). One of the most present negative states in these subjects appears to be determined by anxiety (Mcdowell et al., 2017) . Anxiety, considered an unpleasant state of mind characterized by feelings of apprehension and thoughts of worry, has an estimated prevalence of 31% in patients with FM (Murphy et al., 2012), compared to 4% in the general population (Baxter et al., 2014). Anxiety can be an appropriate response to stressful events and circumstances (Kessler et al., 2007); however, if anxiety persists in the absence and/or when these events and circumstances cease, it may become maladaptive. This type of anxiety is characteristic of individuals suffering from FM but often goes unrecognized and untreated (Mcdowell et al., 2017). This may have a negative effect on treatment outcomes, in part because anxious patients may be less likely to adhere to prescribed medical treatments (Sherbourne et al., 1992). The presence of anxiety symptoms in FM patients has been directly associated with FM pain (Arnold et al., 2006) and physical fitness has been inversely associated with anxiety (Córdoba-Torrecilla et al., 2016). Patients with FM often fear exercise, report that exercise is more painful (Cook et al., 2006), and are significantly less active than the rest of the population (Mcloughlin et al., 2011). This results in very low levels of physical activity among FM patients (Kop et al., 2005) and evidence has demonstrated both associations between low levels of physical activity and anxiety (Stubbs et al., 2017) and increased of anxiety resulting from the consequent increase in sedentary behavior (Edwards & Loprinzi, 2016). Reviews have, on the basis of these associations, researched and summarized the effect of physical exercise on anxiety symptoms among patients with FM (Herring et al., 2010), identifying an improvement in the majority of patients in the different studies (Rossy et al., 1999).

Another characteristic aspect is depression, also listed as one of the main symptoms of FM and the prevalence varies from 20% to 86%, depending on the study (Borchers & Gershwin, 2015). However, this relationship is not well understood, some studies have tried to explain it, in particular one study found that the influence of genetics and environment and the interactions between these can predispose individuals to develop FM and depression (Gracely et al., 2012). It has been shown that 83.3% of patients with FM present clinically significant depressive symptoms; the worse these symptoms were, the higher the scores for pain levels and the lower the quality of life, compared to those without depressive symptoms (Aguglia et al., 2011). Also, in this case the literature reports that physical exercise is important for reducing depressive symptoms in patients with FM. Through a meta-analysis it was possible to verify that aerobic exercise reduces depression scores in these subjects (Häuser et al., 2010); for this reason, aerobic exercise can be considered particularly effective in the treatment of FM, as it is associated with a significant improvement in the average values of functionality, pain, fatigue, rest, stiffness, anxiety, depression and impact on quality of life (Vural et al., 2014). In addition to aerobic exercise, strength training also has positive effects in reducing depressive symptoms. Consequently, significant differences in the reduction of depression were found in groups of patients with FM who performed aerobic exercises or strength training (Bircan et al., 2008).

3.2 Effects of physical activity on pain, flexibility, balance and Quality of Life

As already mentioned, the main clinical manifestation of FM is widespread pain, this can be in combination with the presence of multiple tender points (Wolfe et al., 2016). In addition to pain, fibromyalgia patients may present sensory symptoms, such as paresthesias, motor symptoms, such as muscle stiffness, contractures and tremors, and vegetative symptoms, such as tingling sensations (Rivera et al., 2006).

Several authors have suggested that these symptoms may influence the functional capacity of these patients (Kingsley et al., 2005). This is based on the association between symptoms, flexibility, and balance disorders (Assumpção et al., 2010). Furthermore, balance disorder is a very frequent sign in people suffering from FM and is considered one of the 10 most disabling symptoms, with a prevalence between 45% and 68% (Jones et al., 2009). A study conducted by Jones et al. (2010) showed that people with FM had significantly lower scores on several aspects of balance and fell six times more than healthy subjects. Balance disorders and functional capacity are closely related and have a significant impact on the quality of life of people with FM. According to scientific evidence, these functional deficits in people with FM are related to the level of physical activity performed (Jones et al., 2010).

Several systematic reviews have analyzed the effectiveness of physical exercise programs, alone or in combination with other forms of physical or cognitive intervention (Busch et al., 2007); all concluded that exercise improves the quality of life of these patients.

Complementary and alternative therapies are currently used as a non-pharmacological intervention for the management of FM (Jiao et al., 2019). The World Health Organization defines wellness exercise (Qi Gong) as: "A component of traditional Chinese medicine that combines movement, meditation and regulation of breathing to improve the flow of vital energy (Qi) in the body, for improve circulation and the immune system". Qi Gong is an aerobic exercise, which involves mental concentration, breathing that accompanies the movement, static postures and dynamic movements that combine stretching and activation of the muscle chains through isometric and isotonic contractions; it also includes self-massage movements and work on flexibility, strength, proprioception, coordination and balance (Park et al., 2016). Qi Gong also corrects the posture of the spine and pelvis and prevents energy stagnation in the joints (Ahn et al., 2016). On this basis, scientific research suggests that low-intensity aerobic exercise and meditative movement therapies, such as Qi Gong, are recommended for the treatment of patients with FM, as they improve their symptoms and quality of life (Häuser, 2016).

The study conducted by Rodríguez-Mansilla et al. (2021) demonstrated how an active wellness exercise program improved static balance, flexibility, and pain in women with FM; all the improvements in terms of flexibility and balance have undoubtedly influenced the pain and improvement in the quality of life perceived by patients. Furthermore, Busch et al. (2007) concluded that short-term aerobic exercise in FM patients improves pain, overall sense of well-being, and physical function.

Furthermore, a further study conducted by Yang et al. (2005) showed how a 4-week wellness exercise program helped improve chronic pain and mood disorders in patients with FM.

3.3 Targeted physical activity or non-specific training? Comparison of the effects on Quality of Life

FM is a complex syndrome that includes a wide range of symptoms and functional limitations (Häuser et al., 2015) and reduces quality of life (Perrot et al., 2015). Two factors have been shown to improve quality of life in individuals with FM: diagnosis of the condition and initiation of treatment (Clauw, 2014). Treatment usually involves a multimodal approach, including functional, psychological, pharmacological and socio-professional aspects. The most frequently used non-pharmacological treatments are the following: pain education, cognitive behavioral therapy, composite therapy (education or counseling combined with physical exercise), and aerobic exercise (Häuser et al., 2015).

Exercise has been shown to significantly improve pain and function in individuals with FM (Macfarlane et al., 2017). To date, strength training and aerobic exercise performed dry or as hydrotherapy are equally effective (Bidonde et al., 1996); therefore, current guidelines recommend both aerobic exercise and strength training (Bidonde et al., 2017). The recommended dose of aerobic exercise is 20 minutes (or 10 minutes twice), two to three times per week (at 70-80% of your theoretical maximum heart rate), and eight repetitions of each strengthening exercise two to three times per week (Macfarlane et al., 2017). However, it has been suggested that the dose of exercise should be tailored to the needs of the individual.

FM is a chronic condition and, for chronic medical conditions (Kivelä et al., 2014), in addition to teaching patients to exercise, they must also be taught to manage the condition themselves and to be actively involved in treatment. This is called lifestyle coaching. A pilot study of 10 individuals with FM (Hackshaw et al., 2016) showed a 37% improvement in patient's quality of life by administering a questionnaire following lifestyle coaching sessions with healthcare professionals.

There is ongoing controversy regarding physical therapy for patients with FM. Some groups support it, while others argue that it has the potential to negatively affect FM symptoms, leading to high dropout rates in studies regarding its effectiveness (Harden et al., 2012). Most studies in this field examine the effects of supervised physical therapy. However, in some clinical settings, it may not be possible to supervise groups of patients (or even individual patients) due to a lack of time, facilities, or adequate equipment. Alternative home exercises that patients can perform without supervision may be prescribed. It has yet to be determined which specific type of exercise (aerobic or other) is most effective as therapy for FM.

Physical and manual therapists working in a single-disciplinary clinical setting are often hampered by a lack of time, resources and expertise to conduct supervised exercise programs for patients; therefore, prescribing home exercise programs supervised by **kinesiologists** (see page 179-180) appears to be a better option. Most studies have tended to focus on supervised group exercise as a treatment for FM, while few studies have been conducted to compare the outcomes of home-based exercise for patients with this condition.

A pilot study evaluated the impact of home aerobic conditioning on FM symptoms. A total of 26 sedentary patients with FM undertook a 12-week home aerobic activity regimen (daily exercise for 30 minutes performed at 80% of maximum heart rate/HRmax) at home, outdoors, or in the gym as indicated by the preferences individual of the patient. Subjects who completed the 12-week program demonstrated increased aerobic conditioning and decreased pain. Subjects unwilling or unable to participate in the exercise program appeared to report significantly greater levels of pain and perceived disability, leading to depression, than those who completed the program. The findings indicate that patients with FM who can participate in home aerobic conditioning programs may experience physiological and psychological improvement in their symptoms, particularly in pain ratings. However, those patients who experience significant perceived disability and negative affective symptoms are less likely to maintain a home exercise program and may need a more comprehensive interdisciplinary program that offers a greater degree of social and psychological support (Harden et al., 2012).

3.4 Effects of aquatic and dry land exercise on stress response

Patients with FM show a low level of physical activity compared to healthy people and most of them are sedentary, with a functional capacity like that of elderly people (Pedro Ángel et al., 2012). Furthermore, FM has been associated with a higher prevalence of overweight and obesity compared to the general population. Exercise has been defined as an effective tool for improving the health and quality of life of patients with FM (Kelley & Kelley, 2011). There is much evidence to show that monitored training consisting of aerobic exercises causes beneficial effects on the physical capacity and symptoms of patients with FM, although more studies are needed on the long-term effects of training for increased muscle strength and flexibility (Busch et al., 2008).

Water training and dry training have both been found to have beneficial effects on cardiovascular capacity and daily fatigue (Saltskår Jentoft et al., 2001). A recent meta-analysis (Häuser et al., 2010) showed that there is no evidence to suggest that aquatic aerobic exercise produces comparatively better results than similar dry exercises and established that an aerobic exercise program for patients with FM should consist of water exercise or dry exercise of light to moderate intensity, two to three times per week, for at least four weeks. Few studies have used training programs that combine dry and aquatic exercises (Gowans et al., 2004), demonstrating that this combination of exercises can improve physical function, mood, and symptom severity.

A study conducted by Latorre et al. (2013) aimed precisely at analyzing the effect of a 24-week training program consisting of two weekly sessions of aquatic exercise and one of dry exercise on pain, functional capacity, body composition, and quality of life in women with FM. The results of this study indicated that a 24-week training program (water/dry) with three weekly sessions consisting of muscle strengthening exercises, aerobic resistance, and flexibility reduces pain and improves the impact of the disease, the functional capacity, and quality of life in women with FM. The program was well tolerated and did not cause any adverse health effects on the participants.

A further important finding of the study is that significant improvements were found in the scales of vitality, mental health, social role, and general health of fibromyalgia patients.

These results agree with those of other studies that after 32 weeks of hot water training (three 60-minute sessions per week) found improvements in physical function, body pain, general health, social role, mental health and vitality (Tomas-Carus et al., 2008). Numerous other studies on FM have obtained improvements using therapies consisting of the combination of different physical exercises. However, the overall intervention effect in this study suggests that there may be a positive relationship between aquatic and dry training and muscle strengthening, aerobic endurance, and flexibility.

While many studies have suggested various treatment mechanisms for individuals with FM, few have examined the impact of aquatic and dry exercise on the physiological response to stress in women with FM; Due to the increased physiological and psychological stress associated with FM, further research examining physiological responses to stress and interventions aimed at addressing stress in the population is needed (Kelley & Loy, 2008).

Because there is no known cure, people with FM often feel frustrated with their disease and the many ways it affects their lives.

According to Lazarus and Folkman (1984), stress is a state of anxiety that occurs when events and responsibilities exceed a person's coping abilities. Physiological symptoms of stress often include headaches, sweaty hands, cold extremities, ulcers, diarrhea, hypertension, and a reduction in the ability to fight infections (Romas & Sharma, 2004), all of which can be symptoms associated with FM.

The body's physiological stress response system is activated mainly in the autonomic nervous system and the endocrine system; at the beginning of a stress response, the body prepares for the "battle" by provoking the "fight or flight" response (Cannon, 1939). Individuals exhibiting symptoms of FM are in a constant internal physiological struggle between the sympathetic nervous system and the parasympathetic nervous system (Crofford, 1998).

The sympathetic nervous system of individuals with FM is often overstimulated due to the persistent physical and psychological manifestations of the disease; the endocrine system responds by releasing stress hormones (cortisol) into the bloodstream (Vierck, 2006).

Catley et al. (2000) reported higher baseline cortisol levels, measured in saliva, in individuals with FM compared to healthy controls. It has been suggested that the presence of elevated cortisol levels in healthy individuals is an indicator of increased physiological and/or psychological stress.

Due to the prolonged physiological and psychological distress of individuals affected by FM, anomalies are found in the hypothalamic-pituitary-adrenal axis, the regulatory system of the organism responsible for the secretion of cortisol (Bonifazi et al., 2006).

There are several research studies studying the role of dry aerobic exercise in managing FM symptoms; Martin et al. (1996) suggested that because the fitness of individuals with FM tends to be lower than age- and sex-matched controls, a low-to-moderate exercise program, such as walking, should be included in the FM treatment protocol.

Several researchers have reported that the benefits of a walking program in the fibromyalgia population lead to an improvement in overall physical function, increased self-efficacy, a reduction in sore spots, and an overall improvement in aerobic capacity (Redondo et al., 2004).

Another form of physical activity considered for individuals with FM is aquatic therapy which due to its therapeutic properties has been widely prescribed and administered to individuals with disabilities (Ogden, 2000). Much of the research has focused on aquatic aerobic exercise which has demonstrated positive effects in individuals with FM, such as decreased levels of fatigue, depression, anxiety, pain and stiffness, improved mood, and increased social interaction (Gowens et al., 2001).

A study conducted by Kelley and Loy (2008) aimed to examine the influence of aquatic and dry exercise on the physiological stress response of women with FM; Based on the greater frequency of positive changes in cortisol compared to changes in cortisol concentrations during non-exercise days, both treadmill walking and water exercise demonstrated a positive influence in reducing salivary cortisol in 2/3 of participants. By examining the cortisol response to exercise versus non-exercise days, the results of this study suggested that treadmill exercise conducted at moderate to low intensities had an influence in reducing salivary cortisol concentrations, thus leading to a reduction in the response to perceived physiological or emotional stress.

Both study participants continuously reported high levels of perceived stress in relation to their FM; therefore, by participating in exercise interventions their physiological stress response may have been suppressed (Borer, 2003).

3.5 Physical fitness status in relation to depression, anxiety and Quality of Life

FM is a widespread, painful, debilitating, and psychophysiological chronic disorder that predominantly afflicts middle-aged women and whose etiology remains unknown (Becerra-García & Robles Jurado, 2014). Anxiety and depression are frequent disorders among those who suffer from them (Santos et al., 2012). The symptoms affect every aspect of life and likely contribute to poor physical conditioning. In a treatment program, Carbonell-Baeza et al. (2011) found that a three-month multidisciplinary intervention based on exercises and psychological therapy improved FM symptomatology, including anxiety, depression, and quality of life in women with FM. Furthermore, Guymer et al. (2012) found that the group of FM patients who performed regular exercise had a lower overall disease impact, better physical function, and lower levels of fatigue, anxiety, and depression than those who did not.

FM is often associated with reduced physical function, and physical activity has been recommended to improve global well-being in FM patients. Specialists often advocate the inclusion of leisure-time physical activities (physical training or recreational physical activity) as an important management strategy for individuals with FM (Busch et al., 2008). In FM rehabilitation programs, it is also essential for clinicians to understand and evaluate all aspects of FM patients, including health-related fitness parameters and psychological status. Identifying which health- and performance-related components of physical fitness are impaired and their possible relationships with depression, anxiety, and quality of life in patients with FM may contribute to the development of more beneficial physical rehabilitation strategies.

A study conducted by Sener et al. (2016) specifically wanted to compare VO_2 max, muscle strength, flexibility, daily physical activity, body composition, depression, anxiety and health-related quality of life in patients with FM, for investigate any associations between these parameters; it was discovered that muscle strength, but also the symptoms of depression and anxiety were compromised in patients suffering from FM; anxiety is a significant predictor of the mental component and general health, anxiety and depression symptoms and emotion-focused coping are the most explanatory and most relevant variable symptoms of the impact of FM on quality of life.

FM has a negative impact on patient's quality of life and is known to be strongly associated with depression and anxiety. A detailed evaluation also from a psychological point of view is fundamental for planning and carrying out treatment and rehabilitation (Börsbo et al., 2009). Low muscle strength is often correlated with a reduced quality of life and an increase in depressive and anxious symptoms in patients with FM; suggesting that performing daily exercises that include not only an aerobic component but also strength training as a lifestyle modification may have beneficial effects for patients with FM (Sener et al., 2016).

The prevalence of depression among patients with FM varies from 28.6% to 70% across studies (Epstein et al., 1999). Patients with FM incur large additional healthcare costs in many countries (Sicras-Mainar et al., 2009) and comorbidity of depression in this population is related to greater pain intensity, fatigue, overall disease severity (Soriano-Maldonado et al., 2015) and self-reported affective distress (Thieme et al., 2004), as well as poorer sleep quality and health-related quality of life.

The high prevalence and negative outcomes related to depressive symptoms in patients with FM make it essential to find strategies to improve depressive symptoms in this population.

As a non-pharmacological approach, exercise is becoming increasingly popular for improving physical fitness (Rooks et al., 2004) and improving symptoms of depression (Kelley & Kelley, 2014) and quality of life (Nüesch et al., 2013) in patients with FM.

Physical efficiency is a modifiable multicomponent factor that represents a powerful indicator of health in FM (Soriano-Maldonado et al., 2015) and is closely related to the development of depressive symptoms in the general population (Sui et al., 2009).

Therefore, low levels of physical fitness might be related to high levels of depressive symptoms in women with FM.

The study conducted by Soriano-Maldonado et al. (2016) wanted to detect the relationship between fitness tests carried out in the field and depressive symptoms in women with FM, indicating that better physical fitness is generally associated with less severe depressive symptoms in patients with FM.

Most of the current literature on the relationship between physical fitness and depression focuses on aerobic aspects and muscle strength (Matta Mello Portugal et al., 2013). Gerber et al. (2013) reported that if cardiorespiratory fitness is moderate or high, it has protective effects against depressive symptoms. A large epidemiological study of previously healthy women found that women with moderate or high aerobic capacity had a 46% to 54%

lower chance of incident depression than those with low aerobic capacity (Sui et al., 2009).

It could be hypothesized that low levels of agility (which refers to the ability to move rapidly and change the position of the entire body in space, requiring speed of movement, balance and motor coordination) could have a negative impact on the self-perceived ability to undertake tasks challenging and have a deleterious effect on self-esteem and signs of depression (Petruzzello et al., 1991).

Furthermore, a different association between lower and upper body flexibility with depressive symptoms was observed in patients with FM; although lower body flexibility showed no association with depressive symptoms, upper body flexibility was the primary characteristic that had the strongest association with depressive symptoms. It could be hypothesized that greater flexibility of the upper body could improve the self-perception of the ability to perform activities of daily living, improving the psychosocial level and factors such as self-esteem, social interaction, which are linked to mental health and mood (Peluso & De Andrade, 2005).

References

Aguglia, A., Salvi, V., Maina, G., Rossetto, I., & Aguglia, E. (2011). Fibromyalgia syndrome and depressive symptoms: Comorbidity and clinical correlates. *Journal of affective disorders*, *128*(3), 262–266.

Ahn, Y. J., Jo, S. H., Lee, S. H., & Lim, J. H. (2016). The review study on Yoga, Qigong, and Taichi interventions for anxiety: Based on Korean journal articles from 2009 to 2015. *Journal of Oriental Neuropsychiatry*, *27*(1), 23-31.

Arnold, L. M., Hudson, J. I., Keck, P. E., Auchenbach, M. B., Javaras, K. N., & Hess, E. V. (2006). Comorbidity of fibromyalgia and psychiatric disorders. *Journal of Clinical Psychiatry*, *67*(8), 1219–1225.

Assumpção, A., Sauer, J. F., Mango, P. C., & Marques, A. P. (2010). Physical function interfering with pain and symptoms in fibromyalgia patients. *Clin Exp Rheumatol*, *28*(6 Suppl 63), S57-63.

Baxter, A. J., Scott, K. M., Ferrari, A. J., Norman, R. E., Vos, T., & Whiteford, H. A. (2014). Challenging the myth of an "epidemic" of common mental disorders: Trends in the global prevalence of anxiety and depression between 1990 and 2010. *Depression and anxiety*, *31*(6), 506–516.

Becerra-García, J. A., & Robles Jurado, M. J. (2014). Behavioral approach system activity and self-reported somatic symptoms in fibromyalgia: an exploratory study. *International Journal of Rheumatic Diseases*, *17*(1), 89-92.

Bircan, Ç., Karasel, S. A., Akgün, B., El, Ö., & Alper, S. (2008). Effects of muscle strengthening versus aerobic exercise program in fibromyalgia. *Rheumatology international*, *28*, 527–532.

Bonifazi, M., Suman, A. L., Cambiaggi, C., Felici, A., Grasso, G., Lodi, L., ... & Carli, G. (2006). Changes in salivary cortisol and corticosteroid receptor-α mRNA expression following a 3-week multidisciplinary treatment program in patients with fibromyalgia. *Psychoneuroendocrinology*, *31*(9), 1076-1086.

Borchers, A. T., & Gershwin, M. E. (2015). Fibromyalgia: A critical and comprehensive review. *Clinical reviews in allergy & immunology*, *49*, 100–151.

Borer, K. T. (2003). *Exercise endocrinology*. Human Kinetics.

Börsbo, B., Peolsson, M., & Gerdle, B. (2009). The complex interplay between pain intensity, depression, anxiety and catastrophising with respect to quality of life and disability. *Disability and rehabilitation, 31*(19), 1605-1613.

Busch, A. J., Barber, K. A., Overend, T. J., Peloso, P. M. J., & Schachter, C. L. (2007). Exercise for treating fibromyalgia syndrome. *Cochrane database of systematic reviews*, (4).

Busch, A. J., Schachter, C. L., Overend, T. J., Peloso, P. M., & Barber, K. A. (2008). Exercise for fibromyalgia: a systematic review. *The Journal of rheumatology, 35*(6), 1130-1144.

Busch, A. J., Schachter, C. L., Overend, T. J., Peloso, P. M., & Barber, K. A. (2008). Exercise for fibromyalgia: a systematic review. *The Journal of rheumatology, 35*(6), 1130-1144.

Cannon, W. B. (1939). The wisdom of the body.

Carbonell-Baeza, A., Aparicio, V. A., Chillón, P., Femia, P., Delgado-Fernandez, M., & Ruiz, J. R. (2011). Effectiveness of multidisciplinary therapy on symptomatology and quality of life in women with fibromyalgia. *Clinical and Experimental Rheumatology-Incl Supplements, 29*(6), S97.

Catley, D., Kaell, A. T., Kirschbaum, C., & Stone, A. A. (2000). A naturalistic evaluation of cortisol secretion in persons with fibromyalgia and rheumatoid arthritis. *Arthritis Care & Research, 13*(1), 51-61.

Clauw, D. J. (2014). Fibromyalgia: a clinical review. *Jama, 311*(15), 1547-1555.

Cook, D. B., Nagelkirk, P. R., Poluri, A., Mores, J., & Natelson, B. H. (2006). The influence of aerobic fitness and fibromyalgia on cardiorespiratory and perceptual responses to exercise in patients with chronic fatigue syndrome. *Arthritis & Rheumatism: Official Journal of the American College of Rheumatology, 54*(10), 3351–3362.

Cooney, G. M., Dwan, K., Greig, C. A., Lawlor, D. A., Rimer, J., Waugh, F. R., McMurdo, M., & Mead, G. E. (2013). Exercise for depression. *Cochrane database of systematic reviews*, 9.

Córdoba-Torrecilla, S., Aparicio, V. A., Soriano-Maldonado, A., Estévez-López, F., Segura-Jiménez, V., Álvarez-Gallardo, I., Femia, P., &

Delgado-Fernández, M. (2016). Physical fitness is associated with anxiety levels in women with fibromyalgia: The al-Andalus project. *Quality of Life Research, 25,* 1053–1058.

Crofford, L. J. (1998). The hypothalamic-pituitary-adrenal stress axis in fibromyalgia and chronic fatigue syndrome.

Edwards, M. K., & Loprinzi, P. D. (2016). Experimentally increasing sedentary behavior results in increased anxiety in an active young adult population. *Journal of affective disorders, 204,* 166–173.

Epstein, S. A., Kay, G., Clauw, D., Heaton, R., Klein, D., Krupp, L., ... & Zisook, S. (1999). Psychiatric disorders in patients with fibromyalgia: a multicenter investigation. *Psychosomatics, 40*(1), 57-63.

Gerber, M., Lindwall, M., Lindegård, A., Börjesson, M., & Jonsdottir, I. H. (2013). Cardiorespiratory fitness protects against stress-related symptoms of burnout and depression. *Patient education and counseling, 93*(1), 146-152.

Gowans, S. E., Dehueck, A., Voss, S., Silaj, A., & Abbey, S. E. (2004). Six-month and one-year followup of 23 weeks of aerobic exercise for individuals with fibromyalgia. *Arthritis care & research, 51*(6), 890-898.

Gowans, S. E., DeHueck, A., Voss, S., Silaj, A., Abbey, S. E., & Reynolds, W. J. (2001). Effect of a randomized, controlled trial of exercise on mood and physical function in individuals with fibromyalgia. *Arthritis Care & Research: Official Journal of the American College of Rheumatology, 45*(6), 519-529.

Gracely, R. H., Ceko, M., & Bushnell, M. C. (2012). Fibromyalgia and depression. *Pain research and treatment, 2012.*

Guymer, E. K., Maruff, P., & Littlejohn, G. O. (2012). Clinical characteristics of 150 consecutive fibromyalgia patients attending an Australian public hospital clinic. *International Journal of Rheumatic Diseases, 15*(4), 348-357.

Hackshaw, K. V., Plans-Pujolras, M., Rodriguez-Saona, L. E., Moore, M. A., Jackson, E. K., Sforzo, G. A., & Buffington, C. T. (2016). A pilot study of health and wellness coaching for fibromyalgia. *BMC Musculoskeletal Disorders, 17,* 1-9.

Harden, R. N., Song, S., Fasen, J., Saltz, S. L., Nampiaparampil, D., Vo, A., & Revivo, G. (2012). Home-based aerobic conditioning for management of symptoms of fibromyalgia: a pilot study. *Pain medicine*, *13*(6), 835-842.

Häuser, W. (2016). Fibromyalgia syndrome: Basic knowledge, diagnosis and treatment. *Medizinische Monatsschrift fur Pharmazeuten*, *39*(12), 504-511.

Häuser, W., Ablin, J., Fitzcharles, M. A., Littlejohn, G., Luciano, J. V., Usui, C., & Walitt, B. (2015). Fibromyalgia. *Nature reviews Disease primers*, *1*(1), 1-16.

Häuser, W., Klose, P., Langhorst, J., Moradi, B., Steinbach, M., Schiltenwolf, M., & Busch, A. (2010). Efficacy of different types of aerobic exercise in fibromyalgia syndrome: A systematic review and meta-analysis of randomised controlled trials. *Arthritis research & therapy*, *12*(3), 1–14.

Häuser, W., Klose, P., Langhorst, J., Moradi, B., Steinbach, M., Schiltenwolf, M., & Busch, A. (2010). Efficacy of different types of aerobic exercise in fibromyalgia syndrome: a systematic review and meta-analysis of randomised controlled trials. *Arthritis research & therapy*, *12*(3), 1-14.

Herring, M. P., O'Connor, P. J., & Dishman, R. K. (2010). The effect of exercise training on anxiety symptoms among patients: A systematic review. *Archives of internal medicine*, *170*(4), 321–331.

Jiao, J., Russell, I. J., Wang, W., Wang, J., Zhao, Y. Y., & Jiang, Q. (2019). Ba-Duan-Jin alleviates pain and fibromyalgia-related symptoms in patients with fibromyalgia: results of a randomised controlled trial. *Clinical and experimental rheumatology*, *37*(6), 953-962.

Jones, C. J., Rutledge, D. N., & Aquino, J. (2010). Predictors of physical performance and functional ability in people 50+ with and without fibromyalgia. *Journal of aging and physical activity*, *18*(3), 353-368.

Jones, J., Rutledge, D. N., Jones, K. D., Matallana, L., & Rooks, D. S. (2008). Self-assessed physical function levels of women with fibromyalgia: A national survey. *Women's Health Issues*, *18*(5), 406–412.

Jones, K. D., Horak, F. B., Winters-Stone, K., Irvine, J. M., & Bennett, R. M. (2009). Fibromyalgia is associated with impaired balance and falls. *JCR: Journal of Clinical Rheumatology, 15*(1), 16-21.

Kelley, C., & Loy, D. P. (2008). Comparing the effects of aquatic and land-based exercise on the physiological stress response of women with fibromyalgia. *Therapeutic recreation journal, 42*(2), 103-118.

Kelley, G. A., & Kelley, K. S. (2011). Exercise improves global well-being in adults with fibromyalgia: confirmation of previous meta-analytic results using a recently developed and novel varying coefficient model. *Clinical and Experimental Rheumatology-Incl Supplements, 29*(6), S60.

Kelley, G. A., & Kelley, K. S. (2014). Effects of exercise on depressive symptoms in adults with arthritis and other rheumatic disease: a systematic review of meta-analyses. *BMC Musculoskeletal Disorders, 15*(1), 1-9.

Kessler, R. C., Angermeyer, M., Anthony, J. C., De Graaf, R. O. N., Demyttenaere, K., Gasquet, I., De Girolamo, G., Gluzman, S., Gureje, O. Y. E., & Haro, J. M. (2007). Lifetime prevalence and age-of-onset distributions of mental disorders in the World Health Organization's World Mental Health Survey Initiative. *World psychiatry, 6*(3), 168.

Kingsley, J. D., Panton, L. B., Toole, T., Sirithienthad, P., Mathis, R., & McMillan, V. (2005). The effects of a 12-week strength-training program on strength and functionality in women with fibromyalgia. *Archives of physical medicine and rehabilitation, 86*(9), 1713-1721.

Kivelä, K., Elo, S., Kyngäs, H., & Kääriäinen, M. (2014). The effects of health coaching on adult patients with chronic diseases: a systematic review. *Patient education and counseling, 97*(2), 147-157.

Kop, W. J., Lyden, A., Berlin, A. A., Ambrose, K., Olsen, C., Gracely, R. H., Williams, D. A., & Clauw, D. J. (2005). Ambulatory monitoring of physical activity and symptoms in fibromyalgia and chronic fatigue syndrome. *Arthritis & Rheumatism: Official Journal of the American College of Rheumatology, 52*(1), 296–303.

Latorre, P. A., Santos, M. A., Heredia-Jiménez, J. M., Delgado-Fernández, M., Soto, V. M., Mañas, A., & Carbonell-Baeza, A. (2013). Effect of a 24-week physical training programme (in water and on land) on pain, functional capacity, body composition and quality of life in women with fibromyalgia. *Clin Exp Rheumatol*, *31*(6 Suppl 79), S72-80.

Lazarus, R. S., & Folkman, S. (1984). *Stress, appraisal, and coping*. Springer publishing company.

Macfarlane, G. J., Kronisch, C., Dean, L. E., Atzeni, F., Häuser, W., Fluß, E., ... & Jones, G. T. (2017). EULAR revised recommendations for the management of fibromyalgia. *Annals of the rheumatic diseases*, *76*(2), 318-328.

Martin, L., Nutting, A., MacIntosh, B. R., Edworthy, S. M., Butterwick, D., & Cook, J. (1996). An exercise program in the treatment of fibromyalgia. *The Journal of Rheumatology*, *23*(6), 1050-1053.

Matta Mello Portugal, E., Cevada, T., Sobral Monteiro-Junior, R., Teixeira Guimarães, T., da Cruz Rubini, E., Lattari, E., ... & Camaz Deslandes, A. (2013). Neuroscience of exercise: from neurobiology mechanisms to mental health. *Neuropsychobiology*, *68*(1), 1-14.

Mcdowell, C. P., Cook, D. B., & Herring, M. P. (2017). The effects of exercise training on anxiety in fibromyalgia patients: A meta-analysis. *Medicine & Science in Sports & Exercise*, *49*(9), 1868–1876.

Mcloughlin, M. J., Colbert, L. H., Stegner, A. J., & Cook, D. B. (2011). Are women with fibromyalgia less physically active than healthy women? *Medicine and science in sports and exercise*, *43*(5), 905.

Murphy, L. B., Sacks, J. J., Brady, T. J., Hootman, J. M., & Chapman, D. P. (2012). Anxiety and depression among US adults with arthritis: Prevalence and correlates. *Arthritis care & research*, *64*(7), 968–976.

Nüesch, E., Häuser, W., Bernardy, K., Barth, J., & Jüni, P. (2013). Comparative efficacy of pharmacological and non-pharmacological interventions in fibromyalgia syndrome: network meta-analysis. *Annals of the rheumatic diseases*, *72*(6), 955-962.

Ogden, D. (2000). A different approach for treating fibromyalgia clients in the aquatic environment. *Aquatic Therapy Journal*, *2*, 19-24.

Park, K. S., Jeong, H. Y., & Kim, Y. H. (2016). The effects of Qi-gong exercise on the health of the elderly-with respect to the physical health status, the fear of falling, balance efficacy, and Hwa-Byung. *Journal of Oriental Neuropsychiatry*, *27*(4), 207-214.

Pedersen, B. K., & Saltin, B. (2015). Exercise as medicine–evidence for prescribing exercise as therapy in 26 different chronic diseases. *Scandinavian journal of medicine & science in sports*, *25*, 1–72.

Pedro Ángel, L. R., Campos, M. A. S., Mejía Meza, J. A., Delgado Fernández, M., & Heredia, J. M. (2012). Análise das capacidades físicas de mulheres com fibromialgia segundo o nível de gravidade da enfermidade. *Revista Brasileira de Medicina do Esporte*, *18*, 308-312.

Peluso, M. A. M., & De Andrade, L. H. S. G. (2005). Physical activity and mental health: the association between exercise and mood. *Clinics*, *60*(1), 61-70.

Perrot, S., Vicaut, E., Servant, D., & Ravaud, P. (2011). Prevalence of fibromyalgia in France: a multi-step study research combining national screening and clinical confirmation: The DEFI study (Determination of Epidemiology of FIbromyalgia). *BMC musculoskeletal disorders*, *12*, 1-9.

Petruzzello, S. J., Landers, D. M., Hatfield, B. D., Kubitz, K. A., & Salazar, W. (1991). A meta-analysis on the anxiety-reducing effects of acute and chronic exercise: Outcomes and mechanisms. *Sports medicine*, *11*, 143-182.

Redondo, J. R., Justo, C. M., Moraleda, F. V., Velayos, Y. G., Puche, J. J. O., Zubero, J. R., ... & Pareja, M. Á. V. (2004). Long-term efficacy of therapy in patients with fibromyalgia: a physical exercise-based program and a cognitive-behavioral approach. *Arthritis Care & Research*, *51*(2), 184-192.

Rivera, J., Alegre, C., Ballina, F. J., Carbonell, J., Carmona, L., Castel, B., ... & Vidal, J. (2006). Documento de consenso de la Sociedad Española de Reumatología sobre la fibromialgia. *Reumatología clínica*, *2*, S55-S66.

Rodríguez-Mansilla, J., Mejías-Gil, A., Garrido-Ardila, E. M., Jiménez-Palomares, M., Montanero-Fernández, J., & González-López-Arza, M. V. (2021). Effects of non-pharmacological treatment on pain, flexibility, balance and quality of life in women with fibromyalgia: a randomised clinical trial. *Journal of Clinical Medicine*, *10*(17), 3826.

Romas, J. A., & Sharma, M. (2004). Practical stress management: A comprehensive workbook for managing change and promoting health.

Rooks, D. S., Silverman, C. B., & Kantrowitz, F. G. (2002). The effects of progressive strength training and aerobic exercise on muscle strength and cardiovascular fitness in women with fibromyalgia: a pilot study. *Arthritis Care & Research: Official Journal of the American College of Rheumatology, 47*(1), 22-28.

Rosenbaum, S., Vancampfort, D., Steel, Z., Newby, J., Ward, P. B., & Stubbs, B. (2015). Physical activity in the treatment of post-traumatic stress disorder: A systematic review and meta-analysis. *Psychiatry research, 230*(2), 130–136.

Rossy, L. A., Buckelew, S. P., Dorr, N., Hagglund, K. J., Thayer, J. F., McIntosh, M. J., Hewett, J. E., & Johnson, J. C. (1999). A meta-analysis of fibromyalgia treatment interventions. *Annals of behavioral medicine, 21*(2), 180–191.

Rulleau, T., Planche, L., Etcheverrigaray, F., Dorion, A., Kacki, N., Miot, M., ... & Pluchon, Y. M. (2020). Comparison of patient-led, fibromyalgia-orientated physical activity and a non-specific, standardised 6-month physical activity program on quality of life in individuals with fibromyalgia: a protocol for a randomised controlled trial. *Trials, 21*, 1-11.

Saltskår Jentoft, E., Grimstvedt Kvalvik, A., & Marit Mengshoel, A. (2001). Effects of pool-based and land-based aerobic exercise on women with fibromyalgia/chronic widespread muscle pain. *Arthritis Care & Research: Official Journal of the American College of Rheumatology, 45*(1), 42-47.

Santos, E. B. D., Quintans Junior, L. J., Fraga, B. P., Macieira, J. C., & Bonjardim, L. R. (2012). An evaluation of anxiety and depression symptoms in fibromyalgia. *Revista da Escola de Enfermagem da USP, 46*, 590-596.

Sener, U., Ucok, K., Ulasli, A. M., Genc, A., Karabacak, H., Coban, N. F., ... & Cevik, H. (2016). Evaluation of health-related physical fitness parameters and association analysis with depression, anxiety, and quality of life in patients with fibromyalgia. *International journal of rheumatic diseases, 19*(8), 763-772.

Sherbourne, C. D., Hays, R. D., Ordway, L., DiMatteo, M. R., & Kravitz, R. L. (1992). Antecedents of adherence to medical recommendations: Results from the Medical Outcomes Study. *Journal of behavioral medicine, 15*(5), 447–468.

Sicras-Mainar, A., Rejas, J., Navarro, R., Blanca, M., Morcillo, Á., Larios, R., ... & Villarroya, C. (2009). Treating patients with fibromyalgia in primary care settings under routine medical practice: a claim database cost and burden of illness study. *Arthritis research & therapy, 11*, 1-14.

Soriano-Maldonado, A., Estévez-López, F., Segura-Jimenez, V., Aparicio, V. A., Alvarez-Gallardo, I. C., Herrador-Colmenero, M., ... & al-Ándalus Project. (2016). Association of physical fitness with depression in women with fibromyalgia. *Pain Medicine, 17*(8), 1542-1552.

Soriano-Maldonado, A., Henriksen, M., Segura-Jiménez, V., Aparicio, V. A., Carbonell-Baeza, A., Delgado-Fernández, M., ... & Ruiz, J. R. (2015). Association of physical fitness with fibromyalgia severity in women: the al-Ándalus project. *Archives of Physical Medicine and Rehabilitation, 96*(9), 1599-1605.

Soriano-Maldonado, A., Ruiz, J. R., Aparicio, V. A., Estévez-López, F., Segura-Jiménez, V., Álvarez-Gallardo, I. C., ... & Ortega, F. B. (2015). Association of physical fitness with pain in women with fibromyalgia: the al-andalus project. *Arthritis care & research, 67*(11), 1561-1570.

Stubbs, B., Koyanagi, A., Hallgren, M., Firth, J., Richards, J., Schuch, F., Rosenbaum, S., Mugisha, J., Veronese, N., & Lahti, J. (2017). Physical activity and anxiety: A perspective from the World Health Survey. *Journal of affective disorders, 208*, 545–552.

Stubbs, B., Vancampfort, D., Rosenbaum, S., Firth, J., Cosco, T., Veronese, N., Salum, G. A., & Schuch, F. B. (2017). An examination of the anxiolytic effects of exercise for people with anxiety and stress-related disorders: A meta-analysis. *Psychiatry research, 249*, 102–108.

Sui, X., Laditka, J. N., Church, T. S., Hardin, J. W., Chase, N., Davis, K., & Blair, S. N. (2009). Prospective study of cardiorespiratory fitness and depressive symptoms in women and men. *Journal of psychiatric research, 43*(5), 546-552.

Thieme, K., Turk, D. C., & Flor, H. (2004). Comorbid depression and anxiety in fibromyalgia syndrome: relationship to somatic and psychosocial variables. *Psychosomatic medicine, 66*(6), 837-844.

Thomas, J., Thirlaway, K., Bowes, N., & Meyers, R. (2020). Effects of combining physical activity with psychotherapy on mental health and well-being: A systematic review. *Journal of Affective Disorders*, *265*, 475–485.

Tomas-Carus, P., Gusi, N., Häkkinen, A., Häkkinen, K., Leal, A., & Ortega-Alonso, A. (2008). Eight months of physical training in warm water improves physical and mental health in women with fibromyalgia: a randomized controlled trial. *Journal of rehabilitation medicine*, *40*(4), 248-252.

Vierck Jr, C. J. (2006). Mechanisms underlying development of spatially distributed chronic pain (fibromyalgia). *Pain*, *124*(3), 242-263.

Vural, M., Berkol, T. D., Erdogdu, Z., Pekedis, K., Kuçukserat, B., & Aksoy, C. (2014). Evaluation of the effectiveness of an aerobic exercise program and the personality characteristics of patients with fibromyalgia syndrome: A pilot study. *Journal of physical therapy science*, *26*(10), 1561–1565.

Wolfe, F., Clauw, D. J., Fitzcharles, M. A., Goldenberg, D. L., Häuser, W., Katz, R. L., ... & Walitt, B. (2016, December). 2016 Revisions to the 2010/2011 fibromyalgia diagnostic criteria. In *Seminars in arthritis and rheumatism* (Vol. 46, No. 3, pp. 319-329). WB Saunders.

Yang, K. H., Kim, Y. H., & Lee, M. S. (2005). Efficacy of Qi-therapy (external Qigong) for elderly people with chronic pain. *International journal of neuroscience*, *115*(7), 949-963.

Chapter 4
SPECIFIC EXERCISE PROTOCOLS FOR FIBROMYALGIA SYNDROME

by G. Greco, V. Pugliese, F. Festa, F. Fischetti

4.1 Aerobic activity protocols

People with fibromyalgia (FM) are often intolerant to physical activity and tend to have a sedentary lifestyle which increases the risks of further morbidity (Raftery et al., 2009). Exercise is an important part of managing FM because individuals with FM are often deconditioned by poor physical fitness, cardiovascular endurance (Turk, 2020), muscle strength, and muscular endurance (Bennett & Walczyk, 1998).

It is unclear whether physical deconditioning plays a role in the causal pathway of FM, but several studies have shown that individuals with FM can perform different types of exercise (Carville et al., 2008). Regular exercise is an important factor in counteracting age-related loss of muscle mass, bone mass, and functional independence for the general population; therefore, individuals with FM can improve their overall health and moderate risks associated with other chronic conditions by following an exercise program (Rooks, 2008).

In the different types of activities that can be proposed to subjects with FM, aerobic training can certainly be introduced, the definition of which we have analyzed in the previous chapters given by the guidelines of the American College of Sports Medicine (ACSM, 2013).

The pathophysiology of FM includes changes in brain and neural structure and function, muscle physiology, hormonal factors, neurotransmitters, neuroendocrine transmitters, inflammatory markers, and genetic influences, resulting in increased experience and reduced inhibition of pain and other sensations (Schmidt-Wilcke & Clauw, 2011). Muscle abnormalities that may result in muscle weakness, fatigue, and pain for individuals with FM include reductions in type II fibers, abnormal muscle metabolism, excessive agonist-antagonist co-contraction, reduced adenosine triphosphate levels, and nerve fiber damage (Park et al., 2000). Mood disorders and psychiatric comorbidities, also associated with FM, are linked to disturbed adaptive responses to stress due to abnormalities of the hypothalamic-pituitary axis and interactions between biological, psychological and behavioral mechanisms (Jahan et al., 2012).

Effective treatment and management strategies for FM consist of non-pharmacological therapies such as exercise (Nuesch et al., 2013). It is known that physical exercise, mainly aerobic exercise, increases the feeling of "energy" and improves quality of life and cognitive function (Garber et al., 2011). Regular exercise can also improve experiences of anxiety, depression, and pain and can improve sleep quality (Klaperski et al., 2014).

Aerobic exercise alters neurotransmitters, neuromodulators, brain chemistry, and hypothalamic-pituitary function (Lopresti et al., 2013). These elements are involved in brain function and their improvement through exercise can lead to improved feelings of energy, improved mood and a reduction in stress, anxiety and depression (Moylan et al., 2013). With aerobic exercise, the hypothalamus releases increased levels of neurotransmitters, including endorphins (Barclay et al., 2014). This increase in endorphin release results in a decrease in pain sensation and an improvement in mood states and sleep quality (Yang et al., 2012). Exercise can contribute to pain reduction by improving the physiological response to muscle microtrauma through increased resilience, repair and subsequent adaptation (McLoughlin et al., 2011). Aerobic exercise also leads to a reduction in inflammation and oxidative stress in the body, which results in reduced anxiety and stress responses (Moylan et al., 2013). Overall, aerobic exercise can help improve physiology, which can attenuate changes associated with FM.

Aerobic exercise has been recognized as beneficial to overall health and the prevention/management of chronic conditions for over 50 years (Garber et al., 2011). Growing evidence has demonstrated the benefits of aerobic exercise as a treatment for chronic conditions, including FM (Nunan et al., 2013). Aerobic exercise is the most easily accessible and most recognized form of exercise, making it a reasonable recommendation and treatment strategy (Eyler et al., 2003). Aerobic exercise (e.g., cycling, walking) can be defined as a dynamic physical activity performed using large muscle groups and rhythmic movements that increase heart rate and respiratory rate above resting levels to submaximal levels for a prolonged period (Donatelle & Kolen-Thompson, 2015).

Aerobic exercise protocols for fibromyalgia subjects can include a variable duration between 20 and 24 weeks, with a frequency between two and three times a week, where the average intervention time is 35 minutes (minimum-maximum: from 20 to 60 minutes); the predominant activity may be walking (indoors or outdoors), in some cases it may be accompanied by upper body movements or with a progression towards running. Other modes of aerobic exercise may include activities on a stationary bike, low-impact aerobics activities with music, and rhythmic movements of the lower body muscles (Bidonde et al., 2017).

We can list some examples of aerobic activity protocols for fibromyalgia subjects used in various studies, distinguishing for each the frequency, duration, intensity, and methods of exercises proposed:

- **PROTOCOL 1** (Fontaine et al., 2011)
  Frequency: 5-7 times a week for 12 weeks
  Duration: 60 minutes
  Intensity: Moderate
  Mode: Walking, integrated with other forms of physical activity such as going to do household tasks (gardening, vacuuming) or sporting activities (cycling, swimming).

- **PROTOCOL 2** (Kayo et al., 2011)
  Frequency: 3 times a week for 16 weeks

Duration: 60 minutes (with activation (warm-up) and 5-10 minutes stretching and 5 minutes cooldown)
Intensity: increasing over the weeks, from moderate to vigorous (from 40/50% to 60/70% HRmax)
Mode: Supervised walking indoors or outdoors monitored with a heart rate monitor.

- **PROTOCOL 3** (King et al., 2002)
  Frequency: 3 times a week for 12 weeks
  Duration: initially 10 to 15 minutes and then continuing up to 20-40 minutes
  Intensity: light to moderate (60-75% HRmax)
  Mode: low-impact aerobics walking.

- **PROTOCOL 4 Nordic walking** (Mannerkorpi et al., 2010)
  Frequency: 2 times a week for 15 weeks
  Duration: 20 minutes
  Intensity: 10 minutes light (RPE 9-11), 2 minutes interval moderate to vigorous (RPE 13-15) alternating with 2 minutes light (RPE 10-11)
  Mode: walking in parks and woods with flat areas and hills.

- **PROTOCOL 5** (Ramsay et al., 2000)
  Frequency: once a week for 12 weeks
  Duration: 60 minutes

Intensity: light to moderate

Method: circuit exercises which included STEP-UP, starting from a sitting position and progressing to standing, jumping, jogging on the spot, alternating lateral bends, and circling arms with increasing weights.

- **PROTOCOL 6** (Schachter et al., 2003)

  Frequency: 3 to 5 times a week for 16 weeks

  Duration: 10 to 30 minutes

  Intensity: from moderate in the first week (40/50% HRmax) to vigorous from the tenth week (65/75% HRmax)

  Modality: low-impact aerobics home program with the video-recorded instructor and music, rhythmic movements of the lower body muscles.

- **PROTOCOL 7** (Sencan et al., 2004)

  Frequency: 3 times a week for 6 weeks

  Duration: 40 minutes

  Intensity: Moderate

  Method: aerobic exercise on a cycle ergometer

- **PROTOCOL 8** (Mengshoel et al., 1992)

  Frequency: 2 times a week for 20 weeks

  Duration: 60 minutes

  Intensity: Moderate to vigorous

Method: aerobic dance with upper limb exercises performed at intervals with rest periods, modified to prevent pain, fatigue, and static muscle work.

Finally, there are some APA protocol indications issued in Italy, by the health service of the Tuscany region. This protocol states that the exercise to be performed is aerobic at such an intensity as to be able to speak without difficulty and interruptions while carrying out the activities. Furthermore, you should always work below the perceived pain threshold; the increase in pain and tiredness initially decreases as the treatment continues and can be avoided by introducing breaks in the individual session. At the end of the exercise the patient must feel as if "he could have done more" or rather he must not feel like he is "exhausted" his energy. Therefore, the proposed work must not require excessive energy expenditure, and the pace of the activity must be adapted to the abilities highlighted by the subject. The exercises must always be performed safely to prevent accidents or discomfort during the lesson, including psychological ones.

A typical aerobic training session structure for subjects with FM is shown in Table 4.1 (Häuser et al., 2010).

Table 4.1. Example of an aerobic training session for subjects with fibromyalgia.

Exercise no	Description of exercises	Duration	Material
1. WARM-UP			
1	I walk at various paces and directions or march in place	2-3 minutes	Suitable chairs, parallel or wall bars/bars to support yourself
2	Mobilization of the ankle joints (flexion-extension, circumduction), knee and hip joints (flexion-extension, ab-adduction, circumduction Mobilization of the shoulders (flexion-extension, ab-adduction, circumduction), elbow and wrist (flexion-extension, circumduction)	7-8 minutes	Suitable chairs, parallel or wall bars/bars to support yourself
3	Mobilization of the lumbar and cervical-dorsal spine, pelvis	2 minutes	Suitable chairs, mats
4	Breathing exercise and body perception	2 minutes	Suitable chairs, mats
2. AEROBIC ACTIVITY (UPPER LIMBS)			
5	Active exercises for the shoulder girdle: pectorals, latissimus dorsi, rhomboids	3 minutes	Elastic bands, weights/anklets, sticks
6	Active exercises for the scapulohumeral muscles: teres major, supra and infraspinatus, subscapularis and deltoid	4 minutes	Elastic bands, weights/anklets, sticks
7	Active exercises for the elbow: biceps and triceps brachii	2 minutes	Elastic bands, weights/anklets, sticks
8	Active exercises for the forearm and hand: prone supination of the forearm, opening and closing of the fingers	2 minutes	Elastic bands, weights/anklets, sticks

9	Upper limb stretching	2 minutes	Suitable chairs, mats
2. AEROBIC ACTIVITY (LOWER LIMBS)			
10	Active flexion-extension and hip abduction exercises, with attention to abdominal tightness	4 minutes	Elastic bands, anklets
11	Strengthening exercises for the triceps surae, quadriceps femoris and hamstrings	4 minutes	Elastic bands, anklets, balls
12	Proprioceptive knee and ankle exercises	3 minutes	Elastic bands, anklets, balls
13	I walk at various paces	3 minutes	
14	Stretching of the lower limbs	1 minute	Suitable chairs, mats
3. COOL DOWN			
15	Relaxation techniques combined with breathing, self-massage of the main tender points	7-8 minutes	Suitable chairs, mats
16	Self-correction of posture with body perception techniques	6-7 minutes	Suitable chairs, mats

4.2 Strength (Resistance) training protocols

Most research examining physical activity interventions performed on people with FM has focused on improving cardiorespiratory fitness levels (Saltskår Jentoft et al., 2001). The idea of using strength training to alleviate symptoms appears to have arisen more recently than aerobic protocols, and is probably for this reason a much less used type of intervention, especially in the past (Clark et al., 2001). Strength training has been overlooked as an initial treatment for FM because FM was previously thought to be a direct cause of muscle trauma and that strength training would exacerbate the condition of chronic pain and muscle damage

(Clark et al., 2001). Although research on the effects of strength training in individuals with FM is limited, some studies have shown improvements in strength (Rooks et al., 2002), decreases in total myalgia score (Martin et al., 1996), and decreased impact of FM on everyday life (Rooks et al., 2002). Indeed, the physical deconditioning associated with the pathology leads to an increase in muscular ischemia, increasing peripheral sensitization and thus contributing to central sensitization (Bennett, 1999).

Although the precise etiology of FM is not known, this physical deconditioning is believed to contribute to the development of FM (Busch et al., 1996). Current research, from this point of view, suggests that strength training can slow the deconditioning cycle and allow patients with FM to lead a more "normal" life (Jones et al., 2002).

It has been reported that muscle strength in women with FM is reduced on average by 39% compared to healthy women (Maquet et al., 2002).

Possible physiological explanations for the reduction in strength include structural changes in muscle fibers (Bengtsson, 2002), altered neuromuscular control mechanisms (Gerdle et al., 2010), impaired blood circulation (Elvin et al., 2006), and disturbances in the regulation of growth and energy metabolism (Bennett, 2002). Although muscle deconditioning is known to increase susceptibility to mechanical strain-related microtrauma during physical activities (Bennett, 1993), few studies have evaluated the effects of exercise designed to improve muscle strength in FM (Busch et al., 1996). However, promising effects of strength training on health and pain have been documented, but the paucity of studies implies a low quality of evidence (Busch et al., 1996). One possible reason for the paucity of studies evaluating the effects of strength exercise in FM is the risk of increased pain during isometric muscle contraction (Staud et al., 2005). However, exercise-induced soreness could be avoided by gradually introducing heavier loads (Kristensen & Franklyn-Miller, 2012).

Among strength training, there are exercises defined as "counter-resistance", otherwise called "resistance training", i.e. those workouts that involve lifting one's own body weight or weights, or the use of machines or elastic bands that provide resistance to the movement (Busch et al., 1996). Resistance training has numerous benefits including increased muscle strength, muscle endurance, and muscle power in healthy individuals across the lifespan (Faigenbaum et al., 2009).

Resistance training may be particularly important for protecting individuals from the loss of lean mass and the resulting impairments and activity limitations that occur with aging (Chodzko-Zajko et al., 2009). Furthermore, parameters such as balance, coordination, speed and agility can also be improved with this form of training (Asikainen et al., 2004). The load parameters of these types of workouts, such as intensity and duration, necessary to produce adaptations, depend on a variety of factors, including the fitness level of the individual initiating a resistance training intervention and the desired adaptation.

Typically, neuromuscular adaptations to resistance training are evident within 12 weeks or less in healthy beginners. As the body adapts to a certain stimulus an increase in stimulus is required for further adaptations and improvements. Therefore, if load or volume is not increased over time, progress will be limited. Resistance loading can be applied using various types of equipment (free weights, bands/tubes, weight machines), or simply by using the weight of one or more body segments against gravity to provide resistance.

Training to improve maximum strength (i.e. the ability to generate the maximum possible tension against external resistance) involves the prescription of lower loads, i.e. from 60% to 70% of one repetition maximum (1RM) for beginners and from 80% to 100% of 1RM for more advanced individuals; while a higher number of repetitions (8 to 12 repetitions) is recommended for beginners and fewer repetitions (six repetitions or less) for trained individuals (Garber et al., 2011).

Instead, to improve muscular endurance (i.e., the ability to produce force/tension over time), training involves relatively light loads (40% to 60% of 1 RM) and higher repetitions (15 or more). Training to improve muscle power (i.e., the ability to produce force quickly) involves exercising with light to moderate loads (60% or less of 1 RM) of one to six repetitions at high movement speeds (Busch et al., 1996).

Below are some examples of strength training protocols, used in some of the most relevant studies:

- **PROTOCOL 1** (Bircan et al., 2008)
  Frequency: 3 times a week for 8 weeks
  Duration: 40 minutes
  Intensity: moderate
  Mode: free body in a standing position, sitting or lying down for the muscles of the upper limbs, lower limbs and trunk.

- **PROTOCOL 2** (Häkkinen et al., 2001)
  Frequency: 2 times a week for 21 weeks
  Duration: 60 minutes
  Intensity: progressive moderate to intense (15-20 repetitions at 40-60% of 1 RM progressing to 5-10 repetitions at 70-80% of 1 RM)
  Mode: 6-8 dynamic exercises for the upper and lower limbs and the trunk.

- **PROTOCOL 3** (Jones et al., 2002)
  Frequency: 2 times a week for 12 weeks
  Duration: 60 minutes
  Intensity: Progressed from 4 to 12 repetitions

Method: supervised exercises for the lower and upper limbs and for the trunk with free body or with elastic bands, minimizing eccentric work.

- **PROTOCOL 4** (Kayo et al., 2012)
  Frequency: 3 times a week for 16 weeks
  Duration: 60 minutes
  Intensity: 4 on the RPE scale of 0 to 10, with exercise load and intensity increased every 2 weeks; the training load is individually and systematically adapted every time the participant has successfully performed more than 15 repetitions
  Method: supervised exercise protocol consisting of eleven exercises for the upper, lower limbs and trunk muscles, free body, in an upright position, sitting or lying down.

- **PROTOCOL 5** (Valkeinen et al., 2004)
  Frequency: 2 times a week for 21 weeks
  Duration: 60-90 minutes
  Intensity: light to high, 3 sets of 15-20 repetitions at 40-60% 1RM to 3-5 sets of 5-10 repetitions at 70-80% 1RM
  Modality: dynamic exercises for the knee extensors plus 5-6 exercises for the other main muscle groups.

4.3 Training protocols for flexibility and joint mobility

Many people with FM hesitate to engage in physical activity due to fear of exacerbation of symptoms following exercise, thus potentially increasing the risk of further comorbidities (Nijs et al., 2013). Individuals with FM often experience comorbid conditions, including musculoskeletal conditions, cardiovascular disorders, endocrinological disorders, spondylosis/intervertebral disc disorders and other back problems, irritable bowel syndrome, interstitial cystitis/painful bladder syndrome, chronic pelvic pain, temporomandibular joint disorder, depression, anxiety and other psychiatric disorders. (Ghavidel-Parsa et al., 2015).

Exercise training is now recognized as the cornerstone of FM treatment and management strategies as it represents the strongest evidence available. Non-pharmacological treatments, especially physical training, are recommended as the first treatment option for FM (Macfarlane et al., 2017). Recommendations for treatment of FM include personalized workouts tailored to a person's physical abilities and the level of conditioning in exercises enjoyed or preferred by the individual (Fitzcharles et al., 2013).

Flexibility exercise training is a type of exercise that focuses on improving or maintaining the range of motion of muscles and joint structures by holding or lengthening the body in specific positions (ACSM, 2013). The joint range of motion is an important physical characteristic that influences the ability to perform activities of daily living (Mulholland & Wyss, 2001). Muscle stretching exercises increase the length of the muscle (or muscle group) beyond what would normally be used in normal activity. This can improve the range of motion in as little as 10 sessions with an intensive program (Guissard & Duchateau, 2004).

Different types of stretching exercises can improve the range of motion; ballistic methods use the momentum of the moving body segment to produce elongation, this is commonly used as the activation or warm-up phase (Woolstenhulme et al., 2006).

Dynamic or slow-motion stretching involves a gradual transition from one body position to another, with a progressive increase in range and amplitude of movement as the movement is repeated multiple times (McMillian et al, 2006).

Static stretching involves slowly lengthening a muscle-tendon group while maintaining the position for a period ranging from 10 to 30 seconds for young people and from 30 to 60 seconds for older people (Decoster et al., 2005). Static stretching can be active or passive (Winters et al., 2004); active static stretching involves maintaining the stretching position by exploiting the strength of the agonist muscle. In passive static stretching, you assume a position while holding a limb or other body part with or without the assistance of a partner or device. Static stretching, or maintaining the point of tension or slight discomfort, is the most used stretching modality (Kay et al., 2015). Proprioceptive neuromuscular facilitation (PNF) methods take several forms but typically involve an isometric contraction of the selected muscle-tendon group followed by static stretching of the same group and require assistance from a partner (Rees et al., 2007). Proprioceptive neuromuscular facilitation regularly produces greater increases in range of motion, however, it can be problematic, as performing these contractions can be painful and induce muscle damage (Kay et al., 2015).

Low levels of flexibility have been associated with postural problems, pain, injury, decreased local vascularity and increased neuromuscular tension (Dos Santos Coelho, 2008). Indeed, flexibility training programs have been used to improve a person's well-being and as a tool for symptom management in several clinical populations such as those with major depressive disorders (Ambrose & Golightly, 2015).

The primary goal of flexibility training is usually to improve or maintain the range of motion in major muscle-tendon groups by individualized goals (ACSM, 2013). Flexibility training improves postural stability and balance (Costa et al., 2009), physical function, range of motion, and muscle strength (Jones et al., 2006).

Flexibility training reduces FM symptoms such as pain (Valencia 2009), muscle stiffness (Chen et al., 2011), fatigue, and psychological factors such as anxiety and depression (Lanuez et al., 2011). It can be hypothesized that better flexibility training could also improve the self-perceived ability to perform activities of daily living, and therefore improve psychosocial factors such as depressive symptoms (Soriano-Maldonado et al., 2016) and social interaction, which are linked to mental health and mood (Peluso & De Andrade, 2005). Flexibility training can therefore be useful for both improving fitness and controlling symptoms. Since stiffness and reduced range of motion have been shown to reduce health-related quality of life in individuals with FM, flexibility training may help reduce these physical difficulties thereby improving the quality of life of individuals with fibromyalgia (Valencia et al., 2009).

Flexibility exercises are recommended to the general public as a method to increase or maintain the range of motion of the main joints of the body (such as shoulders, hips, knees, ankles, back, and neck) in order to maintain or improve general physical condition (ACSM, 2013). Because incorporating exercise into one's daily routine is no small endeavor, it is the responsibility of clinicians and researchers to identify whether flexibility training should be undertaken to both improve and maintain physical function in individuals with FM; Flexibility exercise training is commonly recommended in individuals with FM due to its effects on disease symptoms and overall health-related quality of life of patients (Kim et al., 1996).

There are different training protocols which in different studies include exercises for the flexibility of fibromyalgia subjects:

- **PROTOCOL 1** (Altan et al., 2009)
  Frequency: 3 times a week for 12 weeks

Duration: 60 minutes

Intensity: Moderate

Modalities: nine modules regarding postural education, seeking the neutral position, sitting exercises, "pain-relieving exercises" and breathing education. Elastic bands or Pilates balls were used as resistance for the exercises; resistance and stabilization, flexibility and range of motion, correct body alignment, balance, coordination, and body awareness were included in the exercises.

- **PROTOCOL 2** (Amanollahi et al., 2013)

    Frequency: 3 times a week for 4 weeks

    Duration: 40 minutes

    Intensity: light to moderate

    Method: static and non-load stretching with three repetitions of 30 seconds on the scapular muscles, paraspinal muscles, neck muscles and lumbar part of the back, hamstring and calf muscles.

- **PROTOCOL 3** (Assumpcao et al., 2017)

    Frequency: 2 times a week for 12 weeks

    Duration: 40 minutes

    Intensity: in the initial phases 3 repetitions, from the fifth week 4 repetitions, from the ninth week 5 repetitions

Method: relaxation/stretching exercises at home holding the position for 30 seconds, mainly on the triceps surae, gluteal, hamstring, paravertebral, latissimus dorsi, hip adductor and pectoralis muscles.

- **PROTOCOL 4 (**Bressan et al., 2008)

    Frequency: once a week for 8 weeks

    Duration: 40-45 minutes with 5 repetitions of 30 seconds each

    Intensity: moderate

    Modality: static stretches of the triceps surae, ischiotibial, gluteal, paravertebral, pectoralis, trapezius and respiratory muscles.

- **PROTOCOL 5** (Matsutani et al., 2012)

    Frequency: once a week for 8 weeks

    Duration: 45 minutes

    Intensity: light

    Modality: static stretches held for 30 seconds, repeated 4 times with 30 seconds of rest, progressing from lying exercises to sitting and standing, standing or bending, breathing and postural alignment were emphasized in all exercises, using a mirror as an aid for a better perception of movements.

- **PROTOCOL 6** (Calandre et al., 2009)

    Frequency: 3 times a week for 6 weeks

Duration: 60 minutes with 10 minutes of warm-up, 40 minutes of the central phase, and 10 minutes of cool down

Intensity: Dependent on the state of the participant taken into consideration: better physical state greater intensity and vice versa

Method: Active stretching exercises in water, using a wooden stick. Stretching of the trunk muscles, upper and lower atria.

- **PROTOCOL 7** (Valim et al., 2003)

    Frequency: 3 times a week for 20 weeks

    Duration: 45 minutes

    Intensity: 30 seconds of stretching for each position, at maximum stretch

    Mode: 17 different stretching exercises that determined the use of general muscles and joints, including the cervical and extremities of the body

4.4 Combined or multicomponent training

After analyzing the individual types of protocols, we can identify some that refer to "combined" type training, i.e. a series of workouts based on the programmed alternation of multiple activities, a useful element in combating the monotony of training and bringing numerous benefits to general physical preparation; these are exercises that could more commonly be defined as mixed. Training programs with mixed exercises can therefore be identified

with those protocols that include substantial components of at least two of the following types of exercise (Bidonde Torre et al., 2019):
1. aerobic or cardiorespiratory exercise
2. resistance training or muscle strengthening exercise
3. flexibility exercise (excluding all activation and cool-down exercises).

Aerobic exercise activates the cardiovascular and respiratory systems which deliver oxygen to the tissues, allowing an individual to perform sustained work at a given sub-maximal level (ACSM, 2013). Functional capacity can also be improved by resistance training, which improves neuromuscular strength, endurance, or power, depending on the specific exercise prescription. Flexibility exercises affect function by providing the tissues around the joints with a full range of motion (Pollock et al., 1998).

An example of combined or multicomponent training consists in the use of at least two of the three main types of exercises that are mainly used in programs for subjects affected by FM (aerobic, strength, flexibility), specifically combining: aerobic and strength training; aerobic and flexibility; of strength and flexibility; or even combining all three elements of aerobic, strength and flexibility (Bidonde Torre et al., 2019). Each type of exercise should contribute as a significant part of the intervention itself. Other types of exercises, such as those for coordination, balance and relaxation (involving voluntary muscle contractions), have also been considered useful in these types of protocols (Bidonde Torre et al., 2019).

This type of combined training, therefore with mixed exercises, could offer unique advantages, in addition to those derived from interventions that employ only one type of exercise. Individuals would benefit from the adaptive effects associated with multiple forms of exercise (aerobic, strength and flexibility) as they offer the potential to train the cardiorespiratory, vascular and neuro-musculoskeletal systems (Bidonde Torre et al., 2019).

However, to achieve the recommended weekly frequency and duration for each type of exercise (Garber et al., 2011), individuals must dedicate a significant amount of time to exercise; for this reason, exercise professionals may compromise and prescribe lower dosages for each type of exercise to keep the overall program manageable. Certain combinations of exercises have been shown to lead to better results than when programs focus on just one form of exercise. For example, a recent systematic review demonstrated that, in people with type 2 diabetes, combined aerobic and strength training led to improvements in blood glucose and lipid control beyond those achieved with aerobic training. or force conducted in isolation (Schwingshackl et al., 2014). Similarly, combined aerobic and resistance training programs have been shown to result in greater weight and fat loss and improvements in cardiorespiratory fitness among overweight and obese people compared to either program alone (Ho et al., 2012). Although these effects are relevant and important for addressing risk factors and comorbidities common in people with FM (e.g. obesity, low cardiorespiratory fitness, type 2 diabetes), it is not known whether mixed exercise programs have a combined effect on signs and symptoms related to FM. It is possible that combined aerobic and strength training programs may have an additive effect on pain reduction through the release of neurotransmitters centrally and through local muscle adaptations that improve exercise tolerance and allow participants to achieve greater exercise intensities for longer periods of time (Bidonde Torre et al., 2019).

Below are some protocols that have been used in several studies that have treated patients with FM:

- **PROTOCOL 1** (Alentorn-Geli et al., 2008)
  Frequency: 2 times a week for 6 weeks
  Duration: 90 minutes (15-minute warm-up, 30 minutes aerobic activity, 25 minutes flexibility, 20 minutes cooldown)
  Intensity: Moderate to vigorous aerobic activity (65% to 85% of HRmax), flexibility at stopping point
  Method: the aerobic activity part involves walking on flat ground, for flexibility 5x5 stretches of the whole body, 30 seconds of holding, 30 seconds of relaxation, involving the hamstrings, calves, Achilles tendon, shoulders, arms, buttocks, spine, lumbar and dorsal part of the back, thorax, hip adductors.

- **PROTOCOL 2** (Baptista et al., 2012)

    Attendance: Supervised group program twice a week plus an at-home program 2 times a week for 16 weeks

    Duration: 60 minutes supervised program (5 minutes warm up, 45 minutes dance, 15 minutes cool down), 30 minutes home program

    Intensity: Moderate

    Mode: Belly dance (classified by reviewers to be a mixed program including aerobic activity and flexibility).

- **PROTOCOL 3** (Da Costa et al., 2005)

    Frequency: 3 times a week for 12 weeks

    Duration: 60 to 120 minutes per week

    Intensity: Light to moderate (60% to 70% HRMAX) moderate to vigorous (75% to 85% HRmax) aerobic activity, strengthening 12 to 15 bodyweight repetitions, flexibility light stretches held for 15 to 30 seconds for three repetitions

    Modality: Aerobic activity such as walking, swimming, dancing, and water aerobics, for flexibility, static stretches of the upper and lower limbs, isometry for strengthening, and free body exercises for the trunk, upper and lower limbs.

- **PROTOCOL 4** (Demir-Göçmen et al., 2013)

    Frequency: 3 times a week for 12 weeks

    Duration: 60 minutes

Intensity: 10 repetitions for each exercise

Modalities: Flexibility, Balance-coordination-balancing on 1 and 2 feet, partner exercises, push-ups, lateral and backward movements, jumping, rolling.

- **PROTOCOL 5** (Etnier et al., 2009)

  Frequency: 3 times a week for 18 weeks

  Duration: 60 minutes

  Intensity: moderate to vigorous aerobic activity (55% to 65% of HRmax)

  Mode: Aerobic walking activity, 8 stations for strengthening and flexibility.

- **PROTOCOL 6** (Giannotti et al., 2014)

  Frequency: 2 times a week for 10 weeks

  Duration: 60 minutes

  Intensity: Vigorous aerobic activity (70% of HRmax)

  Mode: Flexibility exercises for the spine, upper and lower limbs, strengthening exercises for the lower and upper limbs of 1 set for 10 repetitions, cycle ergometer for aerobic activity.

- **PROTOCOL 7** (Hunt & Bogg, 2000)

  Frequency: Supervised aerobic activity once a week and daily at home; Strengthening once a week supervised and daily at home; Flexibility once a week supervised and daily at home; all repeated for five weeks

Duration: 60 minutes

Intensity: light

Modality: aerobic activity on a stationary bike or STEP UP where patients gradually increase the pace and intensity within their level of perceived effort, 8 core and lower body strengthening exercises (e.g. bridge, push-ups, lateral hip abduction, straight leg raise, lateral hip adduction, isometric abdominal, hip and knee flexion, trunk twist), for flexibility 12 stretches for neck, shoulders, chest, gastrocnemius, hamstrings, where each stretch lasts 5 seconds with 5 repetitions each.

- **PROTOCOL 8** (Jones et al., 2008)

  Frequency: 3 times a week for 26 weeks

  Duration: 60 minutes

  Intensity: light to moderate (10 to 12 on a Borg scale of 6-20)

  Modalities: Low-impact aerobic activity, dynamic strengthening exercises with elastic bands and free weights for all major muscle groups, flexibility through static and dynamic stretching, static and dynamic balance.

- **PROTOCOL 9** (Paolucci et al., 2015)

Frequency: 2 times per week for 5 weeks of supervised group exercise, 2 times per week for 12 weeks of unsupervised home program

Duration: 60 minutes

Intensity: moderate

Method: 20 minutes of low-impact aerobic activity (60% HRmax) through brisk walking in a circle alternating with periods of up and down the stairs, strengthening exercises for the hip and trunk extensors in supine and prone positions, on hands and knees (3 sets of 10 repetitions per exercise), agility and balance exercises, postural exercises for the back and proprioceptive exercises for the trunk in the supine position, diaphragmatic breathing, flexibility exercises with static stretching (shoulders, back muscles of the thigh, quadriceps, gluteus maximus, hip, soleus and gastrocnemius, abdomen, inner thigh) for 30 to 60 seconds repeated 3 times, breathing and relaxation exercises.

- **PROTOCOL 10** (Clarke-Jenssen et al., 2014)

    Frequency: 5 times a week for 4 weeks

    Duration: 115 minutes with a 5-minute warm-up, 45 minutes of aerobic activity chosen from those indicated, 15 minutes of flexibility, 45 minutes of counter-resistance exercises, 5 minutes of cool-down

    Intensity: Low to moderate

Modality: Mixed activity that included daily walking, flexibility training, muscle relaxation exercises (Pilates, etc.), and water exercises (all belonging to the aerobic component) associated with counter-resistance training exercises.

- **PROTOCOL 11** (García-Martínez et al., 2012)
  Frequency: 3 times a week for 12 weeks
  Duration: 60 minutes with 10 minutes aerobic warm-up, 20 minutes aerobic activity, 20 minutes counter-resistance and flexibility activity, 10 minutes cool down
  Intensity: From 60% to 70% of HRmax which can progress up to 75/85% depending on the characteristics of the participants
  Mode: Aerobic and counter-resistance activity not specified.

- **PROTOCOL 12** (Joshi et al., 2009)
  Frequency: Unsupervised home program with flexibility and counter-resistance exercises 2 times a day for 2 days a week; relaxation exercises 2 times a day for 4 days a week and supervised program once a month; for 26 weeks
  Duration: Counter-resistance and flexibility for at least 10 minutes; relaxation exercise for 4 to 6 minutes
  Intensity: Light to moderate
  Modality: Combination of counter-resistance, flexibility and relaxation exercises. Isotonic or isometric counter-resistance

exercises (counter-resistance to gravity); flexibility exercises for the neck, shoulder/scapular girdle.

- **PROTOCOL 13** (Salaffi et al., 2015)
  Frequency: 2 times a week for 12 weeks
  Duration: 60 to 120 minutes per week
  Intensity: From 60% to 85% of HRmax (initially between 60% and 70% and gradually increasing to 75/85%)
  Modality: Combination of aerobic activity, resistance training and flexibility.

- **PROTOCOL 14** (Gentile et al., 2024)
  Frequency: 2 times a week for 12 weeks of supervised home training; from the 12th week to the 48th week, patients were advised to continue following the program, monitoring with monthly telephone interviews
  Duration: 60 minutes with 10 minutes warm-up, 40 minutes aerobic exercise and counter-resistance/muscle strength, 10 minutes cool-down
  Intensity: 1-2 sets with 8-15 repetitions
  Method: Multicomponent home training (aerobic and counter-resistance).

These are just some of the protocols that can be found in reference to combined or multicomponent training linked to fibromyalgia syndrome. The common objective of these training sessions is to determine improvements, which then actually occurred (Bidonde Torre et al., 2019) , relating to some specific parameters such as:

- Health-related quality of life (HRQL) that consists of multidimensional indices used to measure general health status or HRQL, or both (Choy & Mease, 2009)
- Intensity of pain
- Fatigue is recognized by both individuals with FM and clinicians as an important symptom (Choy & Mease, 2009). Fatigue can be measured in a global manner, such as when an individual rates fatigue on a single-item scale, or by using a multidimensional instrument that breaks down the experience of fatigue into two or more dimensions, such as general fatigue, physical fatigue, mental fatigue (Boomershine, 2012)
- Stiffness (Arnold et al., 2008)
- Physical Functioning: this outcome focuses on basic actions and complex activities considered essential for maintaining independence, and those considered discretionary that are not required for independent living, but may impact quality of life (Painter et al ., 1999). Given that cardiorespiratory efficiency, neuromuscular attributes (e.g., muscle strength, endurance, power), and muscle and joint flexibility are

important determinants of physical function, this is a highly relevant finding with respect to interventions using physical exercise (Bidonde Torre et al., 2019).

4.5 Water training protocols

There are therefore several studies that demonstrate how individuals affected by FM can perform different types of exercises such as aerobic, flexibility, and strength training programs (Carville et al., 2008). Despite interest and many new studies, the effects of various types of physical activity on specific symptoms, cognitive functions, and physical performance in people with FM are still unclear.

Furthermore, answers to questions about the best type of exercise, ideal intensity, and additional parameters needed for ideal exercise delivery are still needed.

An attempt may be made to shed light on the effects of water exercise on the well-being, symptoms and fitness of fibromyalgia patients, to guide physicians and exercise professionals in designing the most effective training interventions for this condition (Bidonde et al., 1996).

History shows that baths, spas, water immersions, and natural hot springs were used for religious and healing purposes as early as 2400 BC. The thermal effects of the water were believed to relieve pain and improve relaxation (Geytenbeek, 2002). Also known as pool therapy and hydrotherapy, aquatic exercise is defined by the Chartered Society of Physiotherapists as a therapeutic program designed by a qualified physiotherapist that uses the properties of water to improve function, ideally in a properly heated swimming pool (Zamunér et al., 2019). Balneotherapy refers to the use of hot water treatments to relieve pain, decrease stiffness and relax muscles, and has been further developed with various forms of salt or sulfur (or both) treatments, mud compresses and jets. Water (thermal therapy) (Verhagen et al., 2012).

Healthcare professionals currently use the physical properties of water for the therapy and rehabilitation of a variety of musculoskeletal conditions (e.g., osteoarthritis, rheumatoid arthritis, fractures, tendonitis) (Dagfinrud et al., 2008).

The specific properties of water (buoyancy, resistance, flow and turbulence) are used to develop graded exercise programs. The buoyancy of the body or a body segment, with or without flotation equipment, can be used to assist or resist movement; furthermore, the very viscosity of water provides resistance in all directions. During movement, submerged body parts require greater energy expenditure; this drag can be increased or decreased by altering the speed and directional use of water jets and turbulence.

The intensity of the exercise can also be increased with equipment (e.g., paddles, and webbed gloves) to increase the resistance of the part of the body that moves in the water. Water temperature is another important consideration when designing aquatic exercise training interventions. While most community pools are heated between 26° and 28° Celsius (80° to 84° Fahrenheit) which is pleasantly cool and ideal for movement, pools for therapeutic purposes are usually heated between 30° and 32° Celsius (86° to 90° Fahrenheit) (Bidonde et al., 1996).

Ideally, the use of pharmacological and non-pharmacological therapies is combined in the management of fibromyalgia disease. In this way, non-pharmacological therapies such as an aquatic exercise intervention can be part of a rehabilitation model that addresses core issues such as pain. By combining these therapeutic approaches, pharmacological treatments can help alleviate initial pain symptoms, and aquatic exercise interventions can help address the functional consequences of symptoms.

Therefore, it becomes important to evaluate whether training with aquatic exercises has beneficial effects on the symptoms of FM, how long these effects could last and whether training with aquatic exercises is effective than training with land exercises. It is also important to consider the effects of aquatic exercises as a non-pharmacological treatment, as not all people with FM respond successfully to pharmacological treatment and multimodal treatment types have been shown to be more successful in managing the disease (Rooks et al., 2007).

Different water exercise protocols for subjects with FM used in the various studies can be taken into consideration, specifying the frequency, intensity, duration and methods of the proposed exercises:

- **PROTOCOL 1** (Altan et al., 2004)
  Frequency: 3 times a week for 12 weeks
  Duration: 35 minutes
  Intensity: 60% to 75% of Hrmax
  Modality: flexibility exercises in water with a heated pool and outside the pool, water aerobic activity such as jumping, walking back and forth, and slow swimming.

- **PROTOCOL 2** (Arcos-Carmona et al., 2011)
  Frequency: 2 times a week for 10 weeks
  Duration: 60 minutes (30 minutes in water and 30 minutes dry)
  Intensity: 40% Hrmax
  Mode: Walking, jumping, grabbing and general mobility.

- **PROTOCOL 3** (Assis et al., 2006)
  Frequency: 3 times a week for 15 weeks
  Duration: 60 minutes
  Intensity: 60% to 75% of HRMAX
  Mode: deep water activity in a heated pool (from 28°C to 31°C).

- **PROTOCOL 4** (Calandre et al., 2009)

Frequency: 3 times a week for 6 weeks

Duration: 60 minutes

Intensity: light to moderate

Modality: Tai Chi, patients were taught the 16 movements that constitute tai chi therapy without the aid of any materials, using a combination of deep breathing and slow, sweeping movements of the arms, legs and torso. Stretching in water, performed on the muscles of the main areas of the body: cervical, trunk, upper and lower extremities.

- **PROTOCOL 5** (De Andrade et al., 2008).

    Frequency: 3 times a week for 12 weeks

    Duration: 60 minutes (10 minutes stretching, 40 minutes low impact aerobic activity, 10 minutes cooldown)

    Intensity: between 50% and 75% of Vo2max or between levels 12 and 13 on the Borg Scale 6-20

    Modalities: Supervised aerobic aquatic exercises in the outdoor pool during the summer months, running against water resistance, cycling simulation, stationary walking, bending and extending shoulders and elbows with dumbbells, punches in the air, multidirectional kicks against resistance of the water, pushing and pulling the float against the resistance of the water, stepping and sinking the floats with the feet and Jumping jacks, low jumps using the calf as leverage.

- **PROTOCOL 6** (Gusi et al., 2006)

    Frequency: 3 times a week for 12 weeks

    Duration: 60 minutes (10 minutes of warm-up, 30 minutes of aerobic activity, 20 minutes of strength and 10 minutes of cooldown)

    Intensity: 65% to 75% Hrmax, strength exercises at a very slow pace

    Method: aerobic activity, lower body strength exercises against the resistance of the water (knee flexion and extension).

- **PROTOCOL 7** (Saltskår Jentoft et al., 2001)

    Frequency: 2 times a week for 20 weeks

    Duration: 60 minutes

    Intensity: 60% to 80% of Hrmax

    Modality: supervised program based on an aquatic adaptation of the Norwegian aerobic fitness model with dynamic muscle work accompanied by music (aerobic dance, stretching, strengthening).

- **PROTOCOL 8** (Mannerkorpi et al., 2009)

    Frequency: 1 time a week for 20 weeks

    Duration: 45 minutes

    Intensity: low to moderate

    Modalities: aquatic aerobics, walking, jogging on the flotation device with arm movement, flexibility/coordination, active and passive movements of the arms and trunk, and breathing exercises.

- **PROTOCOL 9** (de Melo Vitorino et al., 2006)
  Frequency: 3 times a week for 3 weeks
  Duration: 60 minutes with 5 minutes of warm-up, 6 minutes of flexibility exercises, 30 minutes of aerobic exercises, 6 minutes of flexibility exercises and 13 minutes of cool down
  Intensity: Light to moderate
  Method: Hydrotherapy exercises in water, with jumping walking, sliding with counter-resistance arm movement.

Below (Table 4.2) is a proposal for water activities following the APA guidelines for fibromyalgia subjects (Langhorst et al., 2009).

Table 4.2. Example of a water activity session for subjects with fibromyalgia.

Exercise no	Description of exercises	Duration	Material
	1. WARM-UP		
1	Gradual setting, vascular route, walking or "cycling" at the edge	2-3 minutes	Low water at the parallel bars
2	Mobilization of the ankle joints (flexion-extension, circumduction), knee and hip joints (flexion-extension, ab-adduction, circumduction Mobilization of the shoulders (flexion-extension, ab-adduction, circumduction), elbow and wrist	7-8 minutes	Low water at the parallel bars

		(flexion-extension, circumduction)		
3		Mobilization of the lumbar and cervical-dorsal spine, pelvis	2 minutes	Low water at the parallel bars
4		Breathing exercise and body perception	2 minutes	Low water at the parallel bars
	2. AEROBIC ACTIVITY (UPPER LIMBS)			
5		Active exercises for the shoulder girdle: pectorals, latissimus dorsi, rhomboids	3 minutes	High water, floating
6		Active exercises for the scapulohumeral muscles: teres major, supra and infraspinatus, subscapularis and deltoid	4 minutes	High water, floating
7		Active exercises for the elbow: biceps and triceps brachii	2 minutes	High water, floating
8		Active exercises for the forearm and hand: prone supination of the forearm, opening and closing of the fingers	2 minutes	High water, floats
9		Upper limb stretching	2 minutes	High water
10		Recovery and relaxation exercises by performing lateral movements with both upper limbs	2 minutes	High water, tablets
	2. AEROBIC ACTIVITY (LOWER LIMBS)			
11		Active flexion-extension and hip abduction exercises, with attention to abdominal tightness	4 minutes	Medium high water, floating
12		Strengthening exercises for the triceps surae, quadriceps femoris and hamstrings	4 minutes	Medium high water, floating
13		Proprioceptive knee and ankle exercises	3 minutes	Medium high water, floating
14		I walk at various paces	3 minutes	Medium high water
15		Stretching of the lower limbs	1 minute	Medium high water
	3. COOL DOWN			
16		Relaxation techniques combined with breathing, self-massage of	7-8 minutes	Medium high water, in

	the main tender points, hydromassage		pairs, tubes, floats
17	Relaxation techniques and perception of the body through floating (also assisted) Gradual emergence to avoid unpleasant "rebound" effects due to the change in temperature	6-7 minutes	Medium high water, in pairs, tubes, floats

4.6 Pilates

In several studies it has been established that exercise programs are useful in patients with FM and in particular programs that include stretching, strength maintenance, and aerobic conditioning have been accepted as a standard treatment protocol (Altan et al., 2004). However, standardization of the type, intensity, and duration of exercise has not yet been delineated and the need for further research on the long-term benefits of physical exercise in FM is highlighted (Busch et al., 2008).

Pilates is a particular approach to physical exercise based on the teachings of Joseph Pilates, initially practiced almost exclusively by athletes and dancers. Pilates has become a popular and rapidly growing trend in rehabilitation and fitness programs in recent years. Pilates can be described as a method that combines Eastern and Western philosophies including yoga, dance, strength training, and gymnastics (Friedman & Eisen, 2005).

The goal of Pilates training is to improve flexibility and overall health of the body by emphasizing core strength, posture, and coordination of breathing with movement (Penelope, 2002). It has been suggested that the Pilates method helps achieve natural flexibility in the spine and limbs by increasing core strength. Although Pilates exercise is generally adopted in training programs for healthy people by fitness professionals, it has been suggested as a therapeutic modality for several musculoskeletal disorders (Levine et al., 2007).

Numerous studies have reported positive results in patients suffering from chronic low back pain who enrolled in Pilates training programs; the positive results have been attributed to the specific training applied to the muscles of the abdomen and the lumbar area of the back, to the consequent increase in the resistance of the spine and to the improvement of the mobility of the joints (Donzelli et al., 2006).

Most patients with FM feel tired and unrested due to the disruption of deep sleep by wake-like bursts of brain activity due to electroencephalographically documented alpha-delta wave intrusions (Hamilton et al., 2008). Therefore, these patients may have difficulty performing standard aerobic exercises. Pilates can be suggested to people with FM because it focuses on isometric contractions and causes less fatigue than aerobic exercises (Altan et al., 2009).

People with FM have muscle asymmetries and antalgic postural problems (Mitani et al., 2006). Jones et al. (2009) demonstrated that FM can influence peripheral and/or central mechanisms of postural control, leading to significantly impaired balance. Johnson et al. (2007) reported an improvement in dynamic balance compared to the control group after ten sessions of Pilates-based exercises.

Pilates exercises can improve impaired posture and balance in patients with FM because Pilates techniques aim to correct body posture by training the muscular system. More specifically, the Pilates concept locates the center of the body in the deep muscles near the spine and the training aims to form a robust musculoskeletal structure in the upper body providing balanced back and abdominal musculature (Muscolino & Cipriani, 2004).

The results of a study conducted by Altan et al. (2009) demonstrated how Pilates exercises had positive effects on the pain and quality of life of fibromyalgia subjects, especially immediately after the exercise program. Although the Pilates method has long been used as part of fitness programs, it has only recently been shown to improve flexibility, abdominal muscle endurance, and static and dynamic balance in healthy people. Subsequently, it became the subject of scientific research which studied its effectiveness in patients with musculoskeletal diseases (Segal et al., 2004).

The fundamental goal of Pilates training is improvement in body flexibility and overall health, with emphasis on core strength, posture and coordination of breathing with movement. Another important contribution of the Pilates technique is the avoidance of positions that require unnecessary muscle recruitment and the consequent early fatigue, decreased stability and compromised recovery (Muscolino & Cipriani, 2004).

Pilates significantly improves pain in FM patients. The mechanisms responsible for the analgesic effect of exercise are not yet clearly understood; Although it is a widely accepted hypothesis that the activation of the endogenous opioid system during exercise plays a key role in the analgesic response mechanism, several researchers have also suggested multiple analgesic system that includes non-opioid mechanisms mediated by other substances such as growth hormone and corticotropin (Ramsay et al., 2000).

The analgesic effect of exercise can also help break the vicious pain-immobility-pain cycle by encouraging patients to participate in exercise programs (Meiworm et al., 2000).

Exercise can also increase patient well-being by preventing muscle hypoxia observed in fibromyalgia patients (Koltyn, 2000).

Subsequently we can observe some examples of Pilates protocols, which have been used in some of the most relevant studies:

- **PROTOCOL 1** (Dias de Aguiar et al., 2016)
  Frequency: 2 times a week for 8 weeks
  Duration: 60 minutes
  Intensity: Moderate
  Method: Various Pilates exercises.

- **PROTOCOL 2** (Altan et al., 2009)
  Frequency: 3 times a week for 12 weeks
  Duration: 60 minutes
  Intensity: Moderate to high
  Method: Various Pilates exercises.

4.7 Tai Chi

Tai Chi is a traditional Chinese exercise that integrates body and mind. It includes breathing control, slow movements, mental relaxation, and meditation. Originating in martial art, the principle of Tai Chi is the appropriate distribution of internal energy, called "qi", throughout the body. With the harmony of "qi" flowing smoothly and powerfully within the body, people can cultivate both physical and mental health (Wayne & Kaptchuk, 2008). Advances in neural technology have also revealed the effects of Tai Chi on anatomical morphologies and neurological activities in the brain (Yu et al., 2018).

Exploratory research has increasingly suggested Tai Chi as a safe exercise to support muscle strength, improve quality of life (QoL), relieve musculoskeletal pain, and alleviate other FM-related syndromes (Geneen et al., 2017). Between 2010 and 2017, five studies (Bongi et al., 2016; Jones et al., 2012; Romero-Zurita et al., 2012; Segura-Jiménez et al., 2014; Wang et al., 2010) involving 36 to 100 subjects with FM, reported benefits (compared to control groups or before/after comparisons) of Tai Chi in the main symptom domains for this condition (pain, sleep, impact, physical function and mental function) (Sawynok, 2018). These studies applied supervised Tai Chi activity and practice sessions two to three times per week for 60 to 90 minutes (one involved additional daily practice at home for 20 minutes), lasted 12 to 28 weeks, and generally used Yang Style Tai Chi (one involved Tai Ji Quan). These studies have uniformly reported health benefits and have been promising (Sawynok, 2018).

In 2018, a comparative study, involving 226 participants with FM, compared the effectiveness of Tai Chi with aerobic exercise (Wang et al., 2018). This was an important study because it compared Tai Chi with the most commonly prescribed non-drug treatment (aerobic exercise); and used well-validated measures (primary outcome measure of the Revised FM Impact Questionnaire, a multidimensional measure of pain, physical function, fatigue, morning tiredness, depression, anxiety, work difficulty, and general well-being); evaluated two Tai Chi regimens (12 or 24 weeks, once or twice a week) and included the recommended home practice of 30 minutes per day; involved long-term follow-up up to 52 weeks. The main findings were as follows: Compared to the control group, the revised Fibromyalgia Impact Questionnaire scores in all five groups were improved; benefits in the combined Tai Chi groups were significantly greater than in the aerobic exercise group in revised Fibromyalgia Impact Questionnaire scores and several secondary outcomes; benefits in the 24-week Tai Chi group compared to the matched intensity and duration of the aerobic exercise group showed significantly greater benefits in the Tai Chi group (Wang et al., 2018).

Participants in all groups decreased their use of analgesic medications by the end of the study, providing further indication of improvements in pain (Wang et al., 2018). In summary, the study reported that both aerobic exercise and Tai Chi produce multiple health benefits in fibromyalgia subjects who have associated comorbidities and poor quality of life, and the findings are of considerable clinical and public health relevance. Baseline characteristics indicated an average pain duration of approximately a decade in each group and multiple drug regimens; The results indicated additional benefits with Tai Chi and exercise, and therefore are important for designing multimodal treatment programs (Sawynok, 2018). Of particular note, with greater benefits observed in the Tai Chi group compared to the matched aerobic exercise group, it appears that Tai Chi involves "something else" besides physical movement and improved fitness.

From a theoretical perspective, given the emerging literature on the health benefits of Tai Chi across many different health areas (Huston & McFarlane, 2016), there is an inherent appeal to a practice that can potentially provide clinical benefits across multiple areas. (Sawynok, 2018).

Below are some protocols that provide a non-pharmacological treatment of FM with the use of Tai Chi:

- **PROTOCOL 1** (Bongi et al., 2016)
  Frequency: 2 times a week for 16 weeks
  Duration. 60 minutes
  Intensity: Light to moderate
  Method: Tai Ji Quan exercises.

- **PROTOCOL 2** (Wong et al., 2018)
  Frequency: 3 times a week for 12 weeks
  Duration: 55 minutes
  Intensity: Moderate
  Method: Tai Chi Yang-style exercises.

4.8 Dance as Movement Therapy

As reiterated, physical exercise is the non-pharmacological therapy with the highest level of evidence in reducing the symptoms of FM (Bidonde et al., 2014) and there are several types of physical exercise that can be used in this area. For example, dance has emerged as a relevant therapy for improving quality of life (Gomes Neto et al., 2014), mortality rate from cardiovascular diseases (Merom et al., 2016), or motivation for physical exercise (Houston & McGill, 2013). In addition to the improvements associated with most types of physical exercise, dance includes rhythmic motor coordination, cognition, emotions, affect, and social interaction (Kattenstroth et al., 2013).

Furthermore, the artistic and creative components lead to further therapeutic benefits due to the integration of the external body with the psychic internal (Purser, 2019). However, different types of dances only involve the repetition of movements and lack the creative, artistic or emotional component. Therefore, it may be possible that the benefits resulting from these types of dances are somewhat limited to the improvements that also result from other physical exercise alternatives (Murillo-Garcia et al., 2018). The artistic and creative concept of dance can be close to the notion of "creative art therapies", which are interventions that use artistic means to approach the participant on a creative level and can have benefits in different types of populations (Martin et al., 2018).

Through dance, patients can perform physical exercise but also develop a sense of self-control, which can lead to a decrease in states of anxiety that can contribute to the development of experiences of stress and pain (Hanna, 1995). Among the types of dances that satisfy the aforementioned concept of artistic and creative dance, we can mention Dance Movement Therapy, Biodance, Aquatic Biodance, or Belly Dance. The American Dance Therapy Association (ADTA) defines Dance Movement Therapy as the psychotherapeutic use of movement to promote the emotional, social, cognitive and physical integration of the participant. Biodance involves movement accompanied by music, inducing experiences capable of modifying the organism on a physiological, affective, motor and existential level (Toro, 1991).

Aquatic Biodance adds the benefits of water-based exercise programs (Gusi & Tomas-Carus, 2008).

Belly dance is an ancient dance form that can promote physical rehabilitation, relaxation, social support, and body-mind connection (Bidonde et al., 2018).

There is evidence describing the benefits of dance for chronic diseases. Dance among individuals with heart failure has demonstrated greater functional and cardiovascular benefits, as well as greater motivation for participation (Kaltsatou et al., 2014) and especially improved quality of life (Gomes Neto et al., 2014) compared to training traditional physique (Bidonde et al., 2017).

Research shows that exercise capacity and quality of life in individuals with Parkinson's disease are improved with dance (Sharp & Hewitt, 2014). Furthermore, dance can improve the locomotor function (i.e. movement from one place to another) of individuals with severe rheumatoid arthritis (Moffet et al., 2000).

Other dance genres such as jazz dance (Alpert et al., 2009), Argentine tango (Pinniger et al., 2012), Turkish folklore (Eyigor et al., 2009), traditional Korean dance (Lee et al., 2013), social dance (Lewis et al., 2016), ballroom dancing (Haboush et al., 2006), modern dance (Lane et al., 2003), waltz (Belardinelli et al., 2008) and Specific dance programs with designed exercises (Vankova et al., 2014) have shown benefits for individuals with a myriad of clinical conditions.

Furthermore, dance promotes greater motivation to exercise (Houston & McGill, 2013), greater attention and cognitive capacity through increased neural connections and blood flow (Alpert, 2011), greater vitality (Koch et al., 2007) and positive effects on mood (Lee et al., 2013), daily skills and social life (Kattenstroth et al., 2013).

Dance can also offer auditory, visual, and sensory stimulation; motor learning; emotional perception; expression; and interaction. All these characteristics make dance an "enriched environment" that stimulates brain plasticity (Kattenstroth et al., 2013).

The characteristics of dance suggest that it is worth evaluating as a means of alleviating FM symptoms (Bidonde et al., 2017).

Below is an example of a dance protocol, applied to individuals with FM:

- **PROTOCOL 1** (López-Rodríguez et al., 2013)
  Frequency: 2 times a week for 12 weeks
  Duration: 60 minutes with 10 minutes of warm-up with flexibility and breathing exercises, 40 minutes of core activity and 10 minutes of cool-down with muscle relaxation exercises
  Intensity: Moderate to high in progression
  Mode: Aquatic Biodance in the pool; activities that include creative dance movements and bodily expressions, associated with interaction and collaboration with other subjects.

References

Alentorn-Geli, E., Padilla, J., Moras, G., Haro, C. L., & Fernández-Solà, J. (2008). Six weeks of whole-body vibration exercise improves pain and fatigue in women with fibromyalgia. *The Journal of Alternative and Complementary Medicine*, *14*(8), 975-981.

Alpert, P. T. (2011). The health benefits of dance. *Home Health Care Management & Practice*, *23*(2), 155–157.

Alpert, P. T., Miller, S. K., Wallmann, H., Havey, R., Cross, C., Chevalia, T., Gillis, C. B., & Kodandapari, K. (2009). The effect of modified jazz dance on balance, cognition, and mood in older adults. *Journal of the American Association of Nurse Practitioners*, *21*(2), 108–115.

Altan, L., Bingöl, U., Aykaç, M., Koç, Z., & Yurtkuran, M. (2004). Investigation of the effects of pool-based exercise on fibromyalgia syndrome. *Rheumatology international*, *24*, 272-277.

Altan, L., Korkmaz, N., Bingol, Ü., & Gunay, B. (2009). Effect of pilates training on people with fibromyalgia syndrome: A pilot study. *Archives of physical medicine and rehabilitation*, *90*(12), 1983–1988.

Amanollahi, A., Naghizadeh, J., Khatibi, A., Hollisaz, M. T., Shamseddini, A. R., & Saburi, A. (2013). Comparison of impacts of friction massage, stretching exercises and analgesics on pain relief in primary fibromyalgia syndrome: a randomized clinical trial. *Tehran University Medical Journal*, *70*(10).

Ambrose, K. R., & Golightly, Y. M. (2015). Physical exercise as non-pharmacological treatment of chronic pain: why and when. *Best practice & research Clinical rheumatology*, *29*(1), 120-130.

American College of Sports Medicine (Ed.). (2013). *ACSM's health-related physical fitness assessment manual*. Lippincott Williams & Wilkins.

Arcos-Carmona, I. M., Castro-Sánchez, A. M., Matarán-Peñarrocha, G. A., Gutiérrez-Rubio, A. B., Ramos-González, E., & Moreno-Lorenzo, C. (2011). Effects of aerobic exercise program and relaxation techniques on anxiety, quality of sleep, depression, and quality of life in patients with fibromyalgia: a randomized controlled trial. *Medicina clínica*, *137*(9), 398-401.

Arnold, L. M., Crofford, L. J., Mease, P. J., Burgess, S. M., Palmer, S. C., Abetz, L., & Martin, S. A. (2008). Patient perspectives on the impact of fibromyalgia. *Patient education and counseling*, *73*(1), 114–120.

Asikainen, T.-M., Kukkonen-Harjula, K., & Miilunpalo, S. (2004). Exercise for health for early postmenopausal women: A systematic review of randomised controlled trials. *Sports medicine*, *34*, 753–778.

Assis, M. R., Silva, L. E., Alves, A. M. B., Pessanha, A. P., Valim, V., Feldman, D., ... & Natour, J. (2006). A randomized controlled trial of deep water running: clinical effectiveness of aquatic exercise to treat fibromyalgia. *Arthritis Care & Research: Official Journal of the American College of Rheumatology*, *55*(1), 57-65.

Assumpcao, A., Matsutani, L. A., Yuan, S. L., Santo, A. S., Sauer, J., Mango, P., & Marques, A. P. (2017). Muscle stretching exercises and resistance training in fibromyalgia: which is better? A three-arm randomized controlled trial. *European journal of physical and rehabilitation medicine*, *54*(5), 663-670.

Baptista, A. S., Villela, A. L., Jones, A., & Natour, J. (2012). Effectiveness of dance in patients with fibromyalgia: a randomized, single-blind, controlled study. *Clin Exp Rheumatol*, *30*(6 Suppl 74), 18-23.

Barclay, T. H., Richards, S., Schoffstall, J., Magnuson, C., McPhee, C., Price, J., ... & Price, J. (2014). A pilot study on the effects of exercise on depression symptoms using levels of neurotransmitters and EEG as markers.

Belardinelli, R., Lacalaprice, F., Ventrella, C., Volpe, L., & Faccenda, E. (2008). Waltz dancing in patients with chronic heart failure: New form of exercise training. *Circulation: Heart Failure*, *1*(2), 107–114.

Bengtsson, A. (2002). The muscle in fibromyalgia. *Rheumatology*, *41*(7), 721–724.

Bennett, R. M. (1993). The origin of myopain: An integrated hypothesis of focal muscle changes and sleep disturbance in patients with the fibromyalgia syndrome. *Journal of musculoskeletal pain*, *1*(3–4), 95–112.

Bennett, R. M. (1999). Emerging concepts in the neurobiology of chronic pain: Evidence of abnormal sensory processing in fibromyalgia. *Mayo clinic proceedings*, *74*(4), 385–398.

Bennett, R. M. (2002). Adult growth hormone deficiency in patients with fibromyalgia. *Current rheumatology reports*, *4*(4), 306–312.

Bennett, R. M., & Walczyk, J. (1998). A randomized, double-blind, placebo-controlled study of growth hormone in the treatment of fibromyalgia. *The American journal of medicine*, *104*(3), 227-231.

Bidonde Torre, M. J., Busch, A. J., Schachter, C. L., Webber, S. C., Musselman, K. E., Overend, T. J., Góes, S. M., Bello-Haas, V. D., & Boden, C. (2019). *Mixed exercise training for adults with fibromyalgia*.

Bidonde, J., Boden, C., Busch, A. J., Goes, S. M., Kim, S., & Knight, E. (2017). Dance for adults with fibromyalgia—What do we know about It? Protocol for a scoping review. *JMIR Research Protocols*, *6*(2), e6873.

Bidonde, J., Boden, C., Kim, S., Busch, A. J., Goes, S. M., & Knight, E. (2018). Scoping review of dance for adults with fibromyalgia: What do we know about it? *JMIR rehabilitation and assistive technologies*, *5*(1), e10033.

Bidonde, J., Busch, A. J., Schachter, C. L., Overend, T. J., Kim, S. Y., Góes, S. M., ... & Cochrane Musculoskeletal Group. (1996). Aerobic exercise training for adults with fibromyalgia. *Cochrane Database of Systematic Reviews*, *2017*(6).

Bidonde, J., Busch, A. J., Webber, S. C., Schachter, C. L., Danyliw, A., Overend, T. J., ... & Cochrane Musculoskeletal Group. (1996). Aquatic exercise training for fibromyalgia. *Cochrane Database of Systematic Reviews*, *2014*(10).

Bidonde, J., Jean Busch, A., Bath, B., & Milosavljevic, S. (2014). Exercise for adults with fibromyalgia: An umbrella systematic review with synthesis of best evidence. *Current rheumatology reviews*, *10*(1), 45–79.

Bircan, Ç., Karasel, S. A., Akgün, B., El, Ö., & Alper, S. (2008). Effects of muscle strengthening versus aerobic exercise program in fibromyalgia. *Rheumatology international*, *28*, 527-532.

Bongi, S. M., Paoletti, G., Cala, M., Del Rosso, A., El Aoufy, K., & Mikhaylova, S. (2016). Efficacy of rehabilitation with Tai Ji Quan in an Italian cohort of patients with Fibromyalgia Syndrome. *Complementary therapies in clinical practice*, *24*, 109–115.

Boomershine, C. S. (2012). A comprehensive evaluation of standardized assessment tools in the diagnosis of fibromyalgia and in the assessment of fibromyalgia severity. *Pain Research and Treatment*, *2012*.

Bressan, L. R., Matsutani, L. A., Assumpção, A., Marques, A. P., & Cabral, C. M. N. (2008). Effects of muscle stretching and physical conditioning as physical therapy treatment for patients with fibromyalgia. *Brazilian Journal of Physical Therapy*, *12*, 88-93.

Busch, A. J., Schachter, C. L., Overend, T. J., Peloso, P. M., & Barber, K. A. (2008). Exercise for fibromyalgia: a systematic review. *The Journal of rheumatology*, *35*(6), 1130-1144.

Busch, A. J., Webber, S. C., Richards, R. S., Bidonde, J., Schachter, C. L., Schafer, L. A., Danyliw, A., Sawant, A., Dal Bello-Haas, V., & Rader, T. (1996). Resistance exercise training for fibromyalgia. *Cochrane database of systematic reviews*, *2014*(7).

Calandre, E., Rodriguez-Claro, M. L., Rico-Villademoros, F., Vilchez, J. S., Hidalgo, J., & Delgado-Rodriguez, A. (2009). Effects of pool-based exercise in fibromyalgia symptomatology and sleep quality: A prospective randomised comparison between stretching and Ai Chi. *Clinical & Experimental Rheumatology*, *27*(5), S21.

Carville, S. F., Arendt-Nielsen, S., Bliddal, H., Blotman, F., Branco, J. C., Buskila, D., ... & Choy, E. H. (2008). EULAR evidence-based recommendations for the management of fibromyalgia syndrome. *Annals of the rheumatic diseases*, *67*(4), 536-541.

Chen, C. H., Nosaka, K., Chen, H. L., Lin, M. J., Tseng, K. W., & Chen, T. C. (2011). Effects of flexibility training on eccentric exercise-induced muscle damage. *Medicine & Science in Sports & Exercise*, *43*(3), 491-500.

Chodzko-Zajko, W. J., Proctor, D. N., Singh, M. A. F., Minson, C. T., Nigg, C. R., Salem, G. J., & Skinner, J. S. (2009). Exercise and physical activity for older adults. *Medicine & science in sports & exercise*, *41*(7), 1510–1530.

Choy, E. H., & Mease, P. J. (2009). Key symptom domains to be assessed in fibromyalgia (outcome measures in rheumatoid arthritis clinical trials). *Rheumatic Disease Clinics*, *35*(2), 329–337.

Clark, S. R., Jones, K. D., Burckhardt, C. S., & Bennett, R. M. (2001). Exercise for patients with fibromyalgia: Risks versus benefits. *Current rheumatology reports*, *3*, 135–146.

Clarke-Jenssen, A.-C., Mengshoel, A. M., Strumse, Y. S., & Forseth, K. O. (2014). Effect of a fibromyalgia rehabilitation programme in warm versus cold climate: A randomized controlled study. *Journal of rehabilitation medicine*, *46*(7), 676–683.

Costa, P. B., Graves, B. S., Whitehurst, M., & Jacobs, P. L. (2009). The acute effects of different durations of static stretching on dynamic balance performance. *The Journal of Strength & Conditioning Research*, *23*(1), 141-147.

Da Costa, D., Abrahamowicz, M., Lowensteyn, I., Bernatsky, S., Dritsa, M., Fitzcharles, M. A., & Dobkin, P. L. (2005). A randomized clinical trial of an individualized home-based exercise programme for women with fibromyalgia. *Rheumatology*, *44*(11), 1422-1427.

Dagfinrud, H., Hagen, K. B., & Kvien, T. K. (2008). Physiotherapy interventions for ankylosing spondylitis. *Cochrane database of systematic reviews*, (1).

De Andrade, S. C., de Carvalho, R. F. P. P., Soares, A. S., de Abreu Freitas, R. P., de Medeiros Guerra, L. M., & Vilar, M. J. (2008). Thalassotherapy for fibromyalgia: a randomized controlled trial comparing aquatic exercises in sea water and water pool. *Rheumatology international*, *29*, 147-152.

de Melo Vitorino, D. F., de Carvalho, L. B. C., & do Prado, G. F. (2006). Hydrotherapy and conventional physiotherapy improve total sleep time and quality of life of fibromyalgia patients: Randomized clinical trial. *Sleep Medicine*, *7*(3), 293–296.

Decoster, L. C., Cleland, J., Altieri, C., & Russell, P. (2005). The effects of hamstring stretching on range of motion: a systematic literature review. *Journal of Orthopaedic & Sports Physical Therapy*, *35*(6), 377-387.

Demir-Göçmen, D., Altan, L. A. L. E., Korkmaz, N. İ. M. E. T., & Arabacı, R. (2013). Effect of supervised exercise program including balance exercises on the balance status and clinical signs in patients with fibromyalgia. *Rheumatology international*, *33*, 743-750.

Dias de Aguiar, S., Paixão Carvalho, J., Andrade Teles, D., & Pôrto, E. F. (2016). Benefício do Método Pilates em mulheres com fibromialgia. *ConScientiae Saude*, *15*(3).

Donatelle, R. J., & Kolen-Thompson, A. M. (2015). Chapter 4: Engaging in physical activity for health, fitness, and performance. *Health: the basics. 6th ed. Toronto: Pearson Canada Inc*.

Donzelli, S., Di Domenica, F., Cova, A. M., Galletti, R., & Giunta, N. (2006). Two different techniques in the rehabilitation treatment of low back pain: a randomized controlled trial. *Europa medicophysica*, *42*(3), 205.

Dos Santos Coelho, L. F. (2008). The muscular flexibility training and the range of movement improvement: a critical literature review/O treino da flexibilidade muscular eo aumento da amplitude de movimento: uma revisao critica da literatura. *Motricidade*, *4*(4), 59-71.

Elvin, A., Siösteen, A.-K., Nilsson, A., & Kosek, E. (2006). Decreased muscle blood flow in fibromyalgia patients during standardised muscle exercise: A contrast media enhanced colour Doppler study. *European journal of pain*, *10*(2), 137–144.

Etnier, J. L., Karper, W. B., Gapin, J. I., Barella, L. A., Chang, Y. K., & Murphy, K. J. (2009). Exercise, fibromyalgia, and fibrofog: a pilot study. *Journal of Physical Activity and Health*, *6*(2), 239-246.

Eyigor, S., Karapolat, H., Durmaz, B., Ibisoglu, U., & Cakir, S. (2009). A randomized controlled trial of Turkish folklore dance on the physical performance, balance, depression and quality of life in older women. *Archives of gerontology and geriatrics*, *48*(1), 84–88.

Eyler, A. A., Brownson, R. C., Bacak, S. J., & Housemann, R. A. (2003). The epidemiology of walking for physical activity in the United States. *Medicine & Science in Sports & Exercise*, *35*(9), 1529-1536.

Faigenbaum, A. D., Kraemer, W. J., Blimkie, C. J., Jeffreys, I., Micheli, L. J., Nitka, M., & Rowland, T. W. (2009). Youth resistance training: Updated position statement paper from the national strength and conditioning association. *The Journal of Strength & Conditioning Research*, *23*, S60–S79.

Fitzcharles, M. A., & Dobkin, P. L. (2005). A randomized clinical trial of an individualized home-based exercise programme for women with fibromyalgia. *Rheumatology, 44*(11), 1422-1427.

Fontaine, K. R., Conn, L., & Clauw, D. J. (2011). Effects of lifestyle physical activity in adults with fibromyalgia: results at follow-up. *JCR: Journal of Clinical Rheumatology, 17*(2), 64-68.

Friedman, P., Eisen, G., & Miller, W. J. (2005). The Pilates Method of Physical and Mental Conditioning Doubleday and Company. *New York*.

Garber, C. E., Blissmer, B., Deschenes, M. R., Franklin, B. A., Lamonte, M. J., Lee, I.-M., Nieman, D. C., & Swain, D. P. (2011). American College of Sports Medicine position stand. Quantity and quality of exercise for developing and maintaining cardiorespiratory, musculoskeletal, and neuromotor fitness in apparently healthy adults: Guidance for prescribing exercise. *Medicine and science in sports and exercise, 43*(7), 1334–1359.

García-Martínez, A. M., De Paz, J. A., & Márquez, S. (2012). Effects of an exercise programme on self-esteem, self-concept and quality of life in women with fibromyalgia: A randomized controlled trial. *Rheumatology international, 32*, 1869–1876.

Geneen, L. J., Moore, R. A., Clarke, C., Martin, D., Colvin, L. A., & Smith, B. H. (2017). Physical activity and exercise for chronic pain in adults: An overview of Cochrane Reviews. *Cochrane Database of Systematic Reviews, 4*.

Gentile, E., Quitadamo, S. G., Clemente, L., Bonavolontà, V., Lombardi, R., Lauria, G., Greco, G., Fischetti, F., & De Tommaso, M. (2024). A multicomponent physical activity home-based intervention for fibromyalgia patients: Effects on clinical and skin biopsy features. *Clinical and experimental rheumatology, 42*, 1156-1163.

Gerdle, B., Grönlund, C., Karlsson, S. J., Holtermann, A., & Roeleveld, K. (2010). Altered neuromuscular control mechanisms of the trapezius muscle in fibromyalgia. *BMC musculoskeletal disorders, 11*, 1–8.

Geytenbeek, J. (2002). Evidence for effective hydrotherapy. *Physiotherapy, 88*(9), 514-529.

Ghavidel-Parsa, B., Bidari, A., Maafi, A. A., & Ghalebaghi, B. (2015). The iceberg nature of fibromyalgia burden: the clinical and economic aspects. *The Korean journal of pain, 28(3)*, 169.

Giannotti, E., Koutsikos, K., Pigatto, M., Rampudda, M. E., Doria, A., & Masiero, S. (2014). Medium-/long-term effects of a specific exercise protocol combined with patient education on spine mobility, chronic fatigue, pain, aerobic fitness and level of disability in fibromyalgia. *BioMed research international, 2014.*

Gomes Neto, M., Menezes, M. A., & Carvalho, V. O. (2014). Dance therapy in patients with chronic heart failure: a systematic review and a meta-analysis. *Clinical Rehabilitation, 28*(12), 1172-1179.

Guissard, N., & Duchateau, J. (2004). Effect of static stretch training on neural and mechanical properties of the human plantar-flexor muscles. *Muscle & Nerve: Official Journal of the American Association of Electrodiagnostic Medicine, 29*(2), 248-255.

Gusi, N., & Tomas-Carus, P. (2008). Cost-utility of an 8-month aquatic training for women with fibromyalgia: A randomized controlled trial. *Arthritis Research & Therapy, 10*, 1–8.

Gusi, N., Tomas-Carus, P., Häkkinen, A., Häkkinen, K., & Ortega-Alonso, A. (2006). Exercise in waist-high warm water decreases pain and improves health-related quality of life and strength in the lower extremities in women with fibromyalgia. *Arthritis Care & Research: Official Journal of the American College of Rheumatology, 55*(1), 66-73.

Haboush, A., Floyd, M., Caron, J., LaSota, M., & Alvarez, K. (2006). Ballroom dance lessons for geriatric depression: An exploratory study. *The Arts in psychotherapy, 33*(2), 89–97.

Häkkinen, A., Häkkinen, K., Hannonen, P., & Alen, M. (2001). Strength training induced adaptations in neuromuscular function of premenopausal women with fibromyalgia: comparison with healthy women. *Annals of the rheumatic diseases, 60*(1), 21-26.

Hanna, J. L. (1995). The power of dance: Health and healing. *The Journal of Alternative and Complementary Medicine, 1*(4), 323–331.

Häuser, W., Klose, P., Langhorst, J., Moradi, B., Steinbach, M., Schiltenwolf, M., & Busch, A. (2010). Efficacy of different types of aerobic exercise in fibromyalgia syndrome: a systematic review and meta-analysis of randomised controlled trials. *Arthritis research & therapy*, *12*, 1-14.

Ho, S. S., Dhaliwal, S. S., Hills, A. P., & Pal, S. (2012). The effect of 12 weeks of aerobic, resistance or combination exercise training on cardiovascular risk factors in the overweight and obese in a randomized trial. *BMC public health*, *12*, 1–10.

Houston, S., & McGill, A. (2013). A mixed-methods study into ballet for people living with Parkinson's. *Arts & health*, *5*(2), 103–119.

Hunt J, Bogg J. An evaluation of the impact of a FM self-management programme on patient morbidity and coping. *Advancing in Physiotherapy 2000*;2(4):168-75.

Huston, P., & McFarlane, B. (2016). Health benefits of tai chi: What is the evidence? *Canadian Family Physician*, *62*(11), 881–890.

Jahan, F., Nanji, K., Qidwai, W., & Qasim, R. (2012). Fibromyalgia syndrome: an overview of pathophysiology, diagnosis and management. *Oman medical journal*, *27*(3), 192.

Johnson, E. G., Larsen, A., Ozawa, H., Wilson, C. A., & Kennedy, K. L. (2007). The effects of Pilates-based exercise on dynamic balance in healthy adults. *Journal of bodywork and movement therapies*, *11*(3), 238-242.

Jones, K. D., & Liptan, G. L. (2009). Exercise interventions in fibromyalgia: clinical applications from the evidence. *Rheumatic Disease Clinics*, *35*(2), 373-391.

Jones, K. D., Adams, D., Winters-Stone, K., & Burckhardt, C. S. (2006). A comprehensive review of 46 exercise treatment studies in fibromyalgia (1988–2005). *Health and quality of life outcomes*, *4*, 1-6.

Jones, K. D., Burckhardt, C. S., Clark, S. R., Bennett, R. M., & Potempa, K. M. (2002). A randomized controlled trial of muscle strengthening versus flexibility training in fibromyalgia. *The Journal of rheumatology*, *29*(5), 1041-1048.

Jones, K. D., Burckhardt, C. S., Deodhar, A. A., Perrin, N. A., Hanson, G. C., & Bennett, R. M. (2008). A six-month randomized controlled trial of exercise and pyridostigmine in the treatment of fibromyalgia. *Arthritis & Rheumatism: Official Journal of the American College of Rheumatology*, *58*(2), 612-622.

Jones, K. D., Clark, S. R., & Bennett, R. M. (2002). Prescribing exercise for people with fibromyalgia. *AACN Advanced Critical Care*, *13*(2), 277–293.

Jones, K. D., Sherman, C. A., Mist, S. D., Carson, J. W., Bennett, R. M., & Li, F. (2012). A randomized controlled trial of 8-form Tai chi improves symptoms and functional mobility in fibromyalgia patients. *Clinical rheumatology*, *31*, 1205–1214.

Joshi, M. N., Joshi, R., & Jain, A. P. (2009). Effect of amitriptyline vs. Physiotherapy in management of fibromyalgia syndrome: What predicts a clinical benefit? *Journal of Postgraduate Medicine*, *55*(3), 185–189.

Kaltsatou, A. C., Kouidi, E. I., Anifanti, M. A., Douka, S. I., & Deligiannis, A. P. (2014). Functional and psychosocial effects of either a traditional dancing or a formal exercising training program in patients with chronic heart failure: A comparative randomized controlled study. *Clinical Rehabilitation*, *28*(2), 128–138.

Kattenstroth, J.-C., Kalisch, T., Holt, S., Tegenthoff, M., & Dinse, H. R. (2013). Six months of dance intervention enhances postural, sensorimotor, and cognitive performance in elderly without affecting cardio-respiratory functions. *Frontiers in aging neuroscience*, *5*, 5.

Kay, A. D., Husbands-Beasley, J., & Blazevich, A. J. (2015). Effects of contract–relax, static stretching, and isometric contractions on muscle–tendon mechanics. *Medicine & Science in Sports & Exercise*, *47*(10), 2181-2190.

Kayo, A. H., Peccin, M. S., Sanches, C. M., & Trevisani, V. F. M. (2012). Effectiveness of physical activity in reducing pain in patients with fibromyalgia: a blinded randomized clinical trial. *Rheumatology international*, *32*, 2285-2292.

King, S. J., Wessel, J., Bhambhani, Y., Sholter, D., & Maksymowych, W. (2002). The effects of exercise and education, individually or combined, in women with fibromyalgia. *The Journal of rheumatology*, *29*(12), 2620-2627.

Klaperski, S., von Dawans, B., Heinrichs, M., & Fuchs, R. (2014). Effects of a 12-week endurance training program on the physiological response to psychosocial stress in men: a randomized controlled trial. *Journal of behavioral medicine, 37*, 1118-1133.

Koch, S. C., Morlinghaus, K., & Fuchs, T. (2007). The joy dance: Specific effects of a single dance intervention on psychiatric patients with depression. *The arts in Psychotherapy, 34*(4), 340–349.

Koltyn, K. F. (2000). Analgesia following exercise: a review. *Sports medicine, 29*, 85-98.

Kristensen, J., & Franklyn-Miller, A. (2012). Resistance training in musculoskeletal rehabilitation: A systematic review. *British journal of sports medicine, 46*(10), 719–726.

Lane, A., Hewston, R., Redding, E., & Whyte, G. P. (2003). Mood changes following modern-dance classes. *Social Behavior and Personality: an international journal, 31*(5), 453–460.

Langhorst, J., Musial, F., Klose, P., & Häuser, W. (2009). Efficacy of hydrotherapy in fibromyalgia syndrome—a meta-analysis of randomized controlled clinical trials. *Rheumatology, 48*(9), 1155-1159.

Lanuez, F. V., Jacob-Filho, W., Lanuez, M. V., & Oliveira, A. C. B. D. (2011). Comparative study of the effects of two programs of physical exercises in flexibility and balance of healthy elderly individuals with and without major depression. *Einstein (São Paulo), 9*, 307-312.

Lee, J. Y., Kim, H. L., & Lim, J. (2013). The effect of korean dance program on climacteric symptoms and blood lipid in rural middle-aged women. *International Journal of Bio-Science and Bio-Technology, 5*(6), 81 90.

Levine, B., Kaplanek, B., Scafura, D., & Jaffe, W. L. (2007). Rehabilitation after Total Hip and Knee Arthroplasty. *Bulletin of the NYU Hospital for joint diseases, 65*(2).

Lewis, C., Annett, L. E., Davenport, S., Hall, A. A., & Lovatt, P. (2016). Mood changes following social dance sessions in people with Parkinson's disease. *Journal of Health Psychology, 21*(4), 483–492.

López-Rodríguez, M. M., Fernández-Martínez, M., Matarán-Peñarrocha, G. A., Rodríguez-Ferrer, M. E., Gámez, G. G., & Ferrándiz, E. A. (2013). Efectividad de la biodanza acuática sobre la calidad del sueño, la ansiedad y otros síntomas en pacientes con fibromialgia. *Medicina Clínica*, *141*(11), 471–478.

Lopresti, A. L., Hood, S. D., & Drummond, P. D. (2013). A review of lifestyle factors that contribute to important pathways associated with major depression: diet, sleep and exercise. *Journal of affective disorders*, *148*(1), 12-27.

Macfarlane, G. J., Kronisch, C., Dean, L. E., Atzeni, F., Häuser, W., Fluß, E., ... & Jones, G. T. (2017). EULAR revised recommendations for the management of fibromyalgia. *Annals of the rheumatic diseases*, *76*(2), 318-328.

Mannerkorpi, K., Nordeman, L., Cider, Å., & Jonsson, G. (2010). Does moderate-to-high intensity Nordic walking improve functional capacity and pain in fibromyalgia? A prospective randomized controlled trial. *Arthritis research & therapy*, *12*, 1-10.

Mannerkorpi, K., Nordeman, L., Ericsson, A., & Arndorw, M. (2009). Pool exercise for patients with fibromyalgia or chronic widespread pain: a randomized controlled trial and subgroup analyses. *Journal of rehabilitation medicine*, *41*(9), 751-760.

Maquet, D., Croisier, J.-L., Renard, C., & Crielaard, J.-M. (2002). Muscle performance in patients with fibromyalgia. *Joint Bone Spine*, *69*(3), 293–299.

Martin, L., Nutting, A., MacIntosh, B. R., Edworthy, S. M., Butterwick, D., & Cook, J. (1996). An exercise program in the treatment of fibromyalgia. *The Journal of Rheumatology*, *23*(6), 1050–1053.

Martin, L., Oepen, R., Bauer, K., Nottensteiner, A., Mergheim, K., Gruber, H., & Koch, S. C. (2018). Creative arts interventions for stress management and prevention—A systematic review. *Behavioral Sciences*, *8*(2), 28.

Matsutani, L. A., Assumpção, A., & Marques, A. P. (2012). Exercícios de alongamento muscular e aeróbico no tratamento da fibromialgia: estudo piloto. *Fisioterapia em Movimento*, *25*, 411-418.

McLoughlin, M. J., Stegner, A. J., & Cook, D. B. (2011). The relationship between physical activity and brain responses to pain in fibromyalgia. *The journal of pain*, *12*(6), 640-651.

McMillian, D. J., Moore, J. H., Hatler, B. S., & Taylor, D. C. (2006). Dynamic vs. static-stretching warm up: the effect on power and agility performance. *The Journal of Strength & Conditioning Research, 20*(3), 492-499.

Meiworm, L., Jakob, E., Walker, U. A., Peter, H. H., & Keul, J. (2000). Patients with fibromyalgia benefit from aerobic endurance exercise. *Clinical Rheumatology, 19,* 253-257.

Mengshoel, A. M., Komnaes, H. B., & Førre, O. (1992). The effects of 20 weeks of physical fitness training in female patients with fibromyalgia. *Clinical and experimental rheumatology, 10*(4), 345–349.

Merom, D., Ding, D., & Stamatakis, E. (2016). Dancing participation and cardiovascular disease mortality: A pooled analysis of 11 population-based British cohorts. *American journal of preventive medicine, 50*(6), 756–760.

Mitani, Y., Fukunaga, M., Kanbara, K., Takebayashi, N., Ishino, S., & Nakai, Y. (2006). Evaluation of psychophysiological asymmetry in patients with fibromyalgia syndrome. *Applied psychophysiology and biofeedback, 31,* 217-225.

Moffet, H., Noreau, L., Parent, E., & Drolet, M. (2000). Feasibility of an eight-week dance-based exercise program and its effects on locomotor ability of persons with functional class III rheumatoid arthritis. *Arthritis Care & Research, 13*(2), 100–111.

Moylan, S., Eyre, H. A., Maes, M., Baune, B. T., Jacka, F. N., & Berk, M. (2013). Exercising the worry away: how inflammation, oxidative and nitrogen stress mediates the beneficial effect of physical activity on anxiety disorder symptoms and behaviours. *Neuroscience & Biobehavioral Reviews, 37*(4), 573-584.

Mulholland, S. J., & Wyss, U. P. (2001). Activities of daily living in non-Western cultures: range of motion requirements for hip and knee joint implants. *International Journal of Rehabilitation Research, 24*(3), 191-198.

Murillo-Garcia, A., Villafaina, S., Adsuar, J. C., Gusi, N., & Collado-Mateo, D. (2018). Effects of dance on pain in patients with fibromyalgia: A systematic review and meta-analysis. *Evidence-Based Complementary and Alternative Medicine, 2018.*

Muscolino, J. E., & Cipriani, S. (2004). Pilates and the "powerhouse"—I. *Journal of bodywork and movement therapies*, *8*(1), 15-24.

Nijs, J., Roussel, N., Van Oosterwijck, J., De Kooning, M., Ickmans, K., Struyf, F., ... & Lundberg, M. (2013). Fear of movement and avoidance behaviour toward physical activity in chronic-fatigue syndrome and fibromyalgia: state of the art and implications for clinical practice. *Clinical rheumatology*, *32*, 1121-1129.

Nüesch, E., Häuser, W., Bernardy, K., Barth, J., & Jüni, P. (2013). Comparative efficacy of pharmacological and non-pharmacological interventions in fibromyalgia syndrome: network meta-analysis. *Annals of the rheumatic diseases*, *72*(6), 955-962.

Nunan, D., Mahtani, K. R., Roberts, N., & Heneghan, C. (2013). Physical activity for the prevention and treatment of major chronic disease: an overview of systematic reviews. *Systematic reviews*, *2*, 1-6.

Painter, P., Stewart, A. L., & Carey, S. (1999). Physical functioning: Definitions, measurement, and expectations. *Advances in renal replacement therapy*, *6*(2), 110–123.

Paolucci, T., Vetrano, M., Zangrando, F., Vulpiani, M. C., Grasso, M. R., Trifoglio, D., ... & Guidetti, L. (2015). MMPI-2 profiles and illness perception in fibromyalgia syndrome: The role of therapeutic exercise as adapted physical activity. *Journal of Back and Musculoskeletal Rehabilitation*, *28*(1), 101-109.

Park, J. H., Niermann, K. J., & Olsen, N. J. (2000). Evidence for metabolic abnormalities in the muscles of patients with fibromyalgia. *Current Rheumatology Reports*, *2*(2), 131-140.

Peluso, M. A. M., & De Andrade, L. H. S. G. (2005). Physical activity and mental health: the association between exercise and mood. *Clinics*, *60*(1), 61-70.

Penelope, L. (2002). Updating the principles of the Pilates method—Part 2. *Journal of Bodywork & Movement Therapies*, *2*(6), 94-101.

Pinniger, R., Brown, R. F., Thorsteinsson, E. B., & McKinley, P. (2012). Argentine tango dance compared to mindfulness meditation and a waiting-list control: A randomised trial for treating depression. *Complementary therapies in medicine*, *20*(6), 377–384.

Pollock, M. L., Gaesser, G. A., Butcher, J. D., Després, J.-P., Dishman, R. K., Franklin, B. A., & Garber, C. E. (1998). ACSM position stand: The recommended quantity and quality of exercise for developing and maintaining cardiorespiratory and muscular fitness, and flexibility in healthy adults. *Journals AZ> Medicine & Science, 30*(6).

Purser, A. (2019). Dancing intercorporeality: A health humanities perspective on dance as a healing art. *Journal of Medical Humanities, 40*(2), 253–263.

Raftery, G., Bridges, M., Heslop, P., & Walker, D. J. (2009). Are fibromyalgia patients as inactive as they say they are?. *Clinical rheumatology, 28*, 711-714.

Ramsay, C., Moreland, J., Ho, M., Joyce, S., Walker, S., & Pullar, T. (2000). An observer-blinded comparison of supervised and unsupervised aerobic exercise regimens in fibromyalgia. *Rheumatology, 39*(5), 501-505.

Rees, S. S., Murphy, A. J., Watsford, M. L., McLachlan, K. A., & Coutts, A. J. (2007). Effects of proprioceptive neuromuscular facilitation stretching on stiffness and force-producing characteristics of the ankle in active women. *The Journal of Strength & Conditioning Research, 21*(2), 572-577.

Romero-Zurita, A., Carbonell-Baeza, A., Aparicio, V. A., Ruiz, J. R., Tercedor, P., & Delgado-Fernández, M. (2012). Effectiveness of a tai-chi training and detraining on functional capacity, symptomatology and psychological outcomes in women with fibromyalgia. *Evidence-based complementary and alternative medicine, 2012*.

Rooks, D. S. (2008). Talking to patients with fibromyalgia about physical activity and exercise. *Current opinion in Rheumatology, 20*(2), 208-212.

Rooks, D. S., Gautam, S., Romeling, M., Cross, M. L., Stratigakis, D., Evans, B., ... & Katz, J. N. (2007). Group exercise, education, and combination self-management in women with fibromyalgia: a randomized trial. *Archives of internal medicine, 167*(20), 2192-2200.

Rooks, D. S., Silverman, C. B., & Kantrowitz, F. G. (2002). The effects of progressive strength training and aerobic exercise on muscle strength and cardiovascular fitness in women with fibromyalgia: A pilot study. *Arthritis Care & Research: Official Journal of the American College of Rheumatology*, *47*(1), 22–28.

Salaffi, F., Ciapetti, A., Gasparini, S., Atzeni, F., Sarzi-Puttini, P., & Baroni, M. (2015). Web/Internet-based telemonitoring of a randomized controlled trial evaluating the time-integrated effects of a 24-week multicomponent intervention on key health outcomes in patients with fibromyalgia. *Clin Exp Rheumatol*, *33*(1 Suppl 88), S93-101.

Saltskår Jentoft, E., Grimstvedt Kvalvik, A., & Marit Mengshoel, A. (2001). Effects of pool-based and land-based aerobic exercise on women with fibromyalgia/chronic widespread muscle pain. *Arthritis Care & Research: Official Journal of the American College of Rheumatology*, *45*(1), 42–47.

Sawynok, J. (2018). Benefits of Tai Chi for fibromyalgia. In *Pain Management* (Vol. 8, Fascicolo 4, pp. 247–250). Future Medicine.

Schachter, C. L., Busch, A. J., Peloso, P. M., & Sheppard, M. S. (2003). Effects of short versus long bouts of aerobic exercise in sedentary women with fibromyalgia: a randomized controlled trial. *Physical therapy*, *83*(4), 340-358.

Schmidt-Wilcke, T., & Clauw, D. J. (2011). Fibromyalgia: from pathophysiology to therapy. *Nature Reviews Rheumatology*, *7*(9), 518-527.

Schwingshackl, L., Missbach, B., Dias, S., König, J., & Hoffmann, G. (2014). Impact of different training modalities on glycaemic control and blood lipids in patients with type 2 diabetes: A systematic review and network meta-analysis. *Diabetologia*, *57*(9), 1789–1797.

Segal, N. A., Hein, J., & Basford, J. R. (2004). The effects of Pilates training on flexibility and body composition: an observational study. *Archives of physical medicine and rehabilitation*, *85*(12), 1977-1981.

Segura-Jiménez, V., Romero-Zurita, A., Carbonell-Baeza, A., Aparicio, V. A., Ruiz, J. R., & Delgado-Fernández, M. (2014). Effectiveness of tai-chi for decreasing acute pain in fibromyalgia patients. *International journal of sports medicine*, *35*(05), 418–423.

Sencan, S., Ak, S., Karan, A., Muslumanoglu, L., Ozcan, E., & Berker, E. (2004). A study to compare the therapeutic efficacy of aerobic exercise and paroxetine in fibromyalgia syndrome. *Journal of Back and Musculoskeletal Rehabilitation, 17*(2), 57-61.

Sharp, K., & Hewitt, J. (2014). Dance as an intervention for people with Parkinson's disease: A systematic review and meta-analysis. *Neuroscience & Biobehavioral Reviews, 47,* 445–456.

Soriano-Maldonado, A., Estévez-López, F., Segura-Jimenez, V., Aparicio, V. A., Alvarez-Gallardo, I. C., Herrador-Colmenero, M., ... & al-Ándalus Project. (2016). Association of physical fitness with depression in women with fibromyalgia. *Pain Medicine, 17*(8), 1542-1552.

Staud, R., Robinson, M. E., & Price, D. D. (2005). Isometric exercise has opposite effects on central pain mechanisms in fibromyalgia patients compared to normal controls. *Pain, 118*(1–2), 176–184.

Turk, D. C. (2020). Suffering and dysfunction in fibromyalgia syndrome. In *The Clinical Neurobiology of Fibromyalgia and Myofascial Pain* (pp. 85-96). CRC Press.

Valencia, M., Alonso, B., Alvarez, M. J., Barrientos, M. J., Ayán, C., & Sánchez, V. M. (2009). Effects of 2 physiotherapy programs on pain perception, muscular flexibility, and illness impact in women with fibromyalgia: a pilot study. *Journal of manipulative and physiological therapeutics, 32*(1), 84-92.

Valim, V., Oliveira, L., Suda, A., Silva, L., de Assis, M., Neto, T. B., Feldman, D., & Natour, J. (2003). Aerobic fitness effects in fibromyalgia. *The Journal of rheumatology, 30*(5), 1060–1069.

Valkeinen, H., Alen, M., Hannonen, P., Häkkinen, A., Airaksinen, O., & Häkkinen, K. (2004). Changes in knee extension and flexion force, EMG and functional capacity during strength training in older females with fibromyalgia and healthy controls. *Rheumatology, 43*(2), 225-228.

Vankova, H., Holmerova, I., Machacova, K., Volicer, L., Veleta, P., & Celko, A. M. (2014). The effect of dance on depressive symptoms in nursing home residents. *Journal of the American Medical Directors Association, 15*(8), 582–587.

Verhagen, A. P., Cardoso, J. R., & Bierma-Zeinstra, S. M. (2012). Aquatic exercise & balneotherapy in musculoskeletal conditions. *Best Practice & Research Clinical Rheumatology, 26*(3), 335-343.

Wang, C., Schmid, C. H., Fielding, R. A., Harvey, W. F., Reid, K. F., Price, L. L., Driban, J. B., Kalish, R., Rones, R., & McAlindon, T. (2018). Effect of tai chi versus aerobic exercise for fibromyalgia: Comparative effectiveness randomized controlled trial. *bmj*, *360*.

Wang, C., Schmid, C. H., Rones, R., Kalish, R., Yinh, J., Goldenberg, D. L., Lee, Y., & McAlindon, T. (2010). A randomized trial of tai chi for fibromyalgia. *New England Journal of Medicine*, *363*(8), 743–754.

Wayne, P. M., & Kaptchuk, T. J. (2008). Challenges inherent to t'ai chi research: Part I—t'ai chi as a complex multicomponent intervention. *The Journal of Alternative and Complementary Medicine*, *14*(1), 95–102.

Winters, M. V., Blake, C. G., Trost, J. S., Marcello-Brinker, T. B., Lowe, L., Garber, M. B., & Wainner, R. S. (2004). Passive versus active stretching of hip flexor muscles in subjects with limited hip extension: a randomized clinical trial. *Physical therapy*, *84*(9), 800-807.

Wong, A., Figueroa, A., Sanchez-Gonzalez, M. A., Son, W.-M., Chernykh, O., & Park, S.-Y. (2018). Effectiveness of tai chi on cardiac autonomic function and symptomatology in women with fibromyalgia: A randomized controlled trial. *Journal of aging and physical activity*, *26*(2), 214–221.

Woolstenhulme, M. T., Griffiths, C. M., Woolstenhulme, E. M., & Parcell, A. C. (2006). Ballistic stretching increases flexibility and acute vertical jump height when combined with basketball activity. *The Journal of Strength & Conditioning Research*, *20*(4), 799-803.

Yang, P. Y., Ho, K. H., Chen, H. C., & Chien, M. Y. (2012). Exercise training improves sleep quality in middle-aged and older adults with sleep problems: a systematic review. *Journal of physiotherapy*, *58*(3), 157-163.

Yu, A. P., Tam, B. T., Lai, C. W., Yu, D. S., Woo, J., Chung, K.-F., Hui, S. S., Liu, J. Y., Wei, G. X., & Siu, P. M. (2018). Revealing the neural mechanisms underlying the beneficial effects of Tai Chi: A neuroimaging perspective. *The American journal of Chinese medicine*, *46*(02), 231–259.

Zamunér, A. R., Andrade, C. P., Arca, E. A., & Avila, M. A. (2019). Impact of water therapy on pain management in patients with fibromyalgia: current perspectives. *Journal of Pain Research*, 1971-2007.

Chapter 5
GUIDELINES FOR EXERCISE PRESCRIPTION AND PRACTICAL APPLICATIONS

by G. Greco, F. Festa, V. Pugliese, F. Fischetti

5.1 Training Programming: Theory and Applications

Regarding the prescription of physical exercise, it is necessary to specify that there is a planning process on its basis. Training planning is an act of systematic structuring of the entire training process based on practical experiences and scientific knowledge, which aims to achieve an athletic goal while respecting the individual's performance level (Martin et al., 1997).

Programming, therefore, is essential to determine the training process itself; specifically, training is defined as the process that tends to improve the respective set objectives (Martin et al., 1997).

The concept of training is closely related to that of physical activity and exercise. In particular, physical activity can be adapted to the needs of different subjects; thus, the concept of Adapted Physical Activity (APA) was born.

The APA refers to all physical exercise programs created for frail individuals with specific needs because they are disabled, ill, or elderly. This term was introduced in 1973, the year the International Federation of Adapted Physical Activity was founded. The protocols are created for people with chronic diseases in a stable situation and have as their main aim that of modifying lifestyle to maintain and improve the state of health and to prevent any worsening linked to a sedentary lifestyle (Farinella et al., 2016).

As evident from the scientific literature, a physically active lifestyle that meets or exceeds minimum recommendations for physical activity confers numerous health-related benefits (Eijsvogels & Thompson, 2015; Lundqvist et al., 2017). Even an initial commitment to levels lower than those recommended induces health benefits (Wen et al., 2011), as does a reduction in the amount of sedentary activity (Same et al., 2016). Although it is not possible to completely prevent all known chronic non-communicable diseases, it is certainly possible to delay their onset by reducing a sedentary lifestyle and practicing regular exercise and physical activity.

To this end, the World Health Organization (WHO, 2020) has provided guidelines for physical activity with specific recommendations for different age groups and population groups. Here are the main recommendations:

- Children and adolescents (5-17 years)

- At least 60 minutes a day of moderate or vigorous intensity physical activity, mainly aerobic.

- At least 3 times a week include activities that strengthen muscles and bones.

- Adults (18-64 years)

- 150-300 minutes per week of moderate-intensity aerobic activity, or 75-150 minutes per week of vigorous aerobic activity, or an equivalent combination.

- At least 2 times a week, including muscle-strengthening activities that involve the main muscle groups.

- Elderly (>65 years)

- Same recommendations as adults, with the addition of physical activities that improve balance and prevent falls, at least 3 times a week.

- People with chronic conditions or disabilities

- Follow the same recommendations as adults, adapting the intensity and type of activity to your abilities and health conditions.

These guidelines highlight the importance of reducing sedentary behaviors and integrating physical activity into your daily routine to improve overall health (Bull et al., 2020). For example, improving cardiorespiratory efficiency or physical fitness promotes biological mechanisms that favorably influence glycemia and lipids, insulin sensitivity, body composition, and cognitive function (Coombes et al., 2015). Similarly, sedentary behavior, defined as an energy expenditure of 1.5 METs, is thought to be a cardiovascular risk factor independent of physical activity levels (Same et al., 2016).

The ACSM created the "Exercise is Medicine (EIM)" initiative to convince physicians and healthcare professionals to include physical activity in the treatment plans prescribed for their patients. Coombes et al. (2015) describe a six-step approach. Overall, this approach revolves around growing awareness of the importance of a physically active lifestyle, appropriately referring patients to qualified exercise professionals i.e. kinesiologists. The **profession of kinesiologist**, a figure with a degree in at least one of the degree courses in Physical Education, was established and regulated in Italy by art. 41 of Legislative Decree 28 February 2021, n. 36, implementing the art. 5 of Law 8 August 2019, n. 86; it is divided into the professional figures of the basic kinesiologist, the kinesiologist of preventive and adapted physical activities, the sports kinesiologist, and the sports manager.

Exercise can reduce symptoms and improve functional capacity and disease-related outcomes. To that end, this chapter provides the necessary guidance and skills a kinesiologist needs to develop and implement safe and effective exercise prescriptions.

An exercise prescription is a specific guidance given to an individual for executing an exercise program.

Despite the use of the term "prescription," developing an exercise prescription does not necessarily require a doctor's approval. In some situations, however, it may require it, especially when the prescription is developed for a patient with a clinically manifest disease or disorder (Pescatello et al., 2004).

Individuals tasked with developing an exercise prescription often find that doing so is both an art and a science; they must possess the necessary knowledge and skills and must be able to articulate and implement a safe and practical prescription.

The primary purpose of exercise prescription is to provide sound and safe guidance for optimal health and improvements in physical efficiency. The specificity of the exercise prescription should be tailored to the nature of the clinical population (Garber et al., 2011).

The American College of Sports Medicine (www.acsm.org/education-resources) has published Position Stands on diverse populations, including healthy people and those with coronary heart disease, osteoporosis, hypertension, and diabetes, as well as older people. Exercise prescription primarily addresses the five health-related components of physical fitness:

1. Cardiovascular Fitness or Cardiorespiratory Endurance: The ability of the cardiorespiratory system to transport oxygen for skeletal muscle activity during prolonged submaximal exercise and the ability of skeletal muscles to utilize oxygen through metabolic pathways. It can be measured by direct testing of VO_2 max.

2. Muscle Strength: the ability of a muscle or muscle group to exert force against resistance. It can be assessed through exercises that involve lifting a load and measured by the one repetition maximum (1RM) test.

3. Muscular endurance: ability to produce submaximal force for a prolonged period. It is measured through low-load resistance exercises.

4. Flexibility: the ability of a joint to move through its full range of motion. It is measured for the lower limbs using the sit and reach test.

5. Body composition: the proportion of body fat to lean mass (muscle, bone, water, etc.). It is evaluated through methods such as the skinfold test, bioimpedance measurement (BIA) or DEXA (Dual-Energy X-ray Absorptiometry).

Each of these components of physical fitness is related to at least one aspect of health, and each component is positively influenced by physical training, possibly reducing the risk of a primary or secondary chronic disease (ACSM, 2017).

Therefore, the importance of regular exercise and physical activity for overall health is well established. The general benefits of regular exercise are as follows (Ehrman et al., 2023):

- Cardiorespiratory and musculoskeletal improvement
- Reduced risk of obesity fitness
- Metabolic, endocrine, and immune improvement
- Overall improvement in health-related quality of life function
- Reduced mortality from all causes
- Reduced risk of cardiovascular disease
- Reduced risk of some cancers (e.g., colon, breast)
- Reduced risk of osteoporosis and arthritis
- Improved health behavior
- Reduced risk of non-insulin-dependent diabetes
- Improved glucose metabolism
- Reduced risk of falling
- Improved sleep rhythm

Furthermore, the kinesiologist must also consider several aspects of a person's psychosocial conditions, such as those relevant to initiating and adhering to a physical training program (Ehrman et al., 2023).

The art of exercise prescribing involves the successful integration of exercise science with behavioral techniques in a way that ensures long-term program compliance and achievement of individual goals. Unlike disciplines such as chemistry or physics, physiology, and psychology are not always exact (Ehrman et al., 2023).

We cannot always accurately predict physiological or psychological responses because numerous factors, including confounding factors, can influence the outcome. These include but are not limited to, age, physical and environmental conditions, gender, previous experience, genetics, and nutrition. When developing an exercise prescription, you need to follow basic guidelines. This can help achieve the desired response both during a single training session and throughout an extended training period. It should be kept in mind, however, that not all people respond as expected, especially those with chronic diseases (Ehrman et al., 2023).

The ACSM lists several reasons for changing exercise prescription in selected individuals:

- Change in objective (physiological) and subjective (perceptual) responses to exercise training
- Change in quantity and rate of responses to training
- Differences in goals between individuals

- Variance in behavioral changes compared to exercise prescription

Each of these reasons should be considered for both the initial development and subsequent revision of the exercise prescription. A modified exercise prescription should not be considered adequate unless its effectiveness over time is evaluated. Typically, a person's exercise prescription should be reevaluated weekly until its parameters appear safe and adequate to improve selected health behaviors and physiological indices (ACSM, 2017).

A complete training program should include flexibility, strength, and cardiorespiratory (aerobic) exercises. The order of your exercise routine is important for both safety and effectiveness.

In general, to develop or maintain full range of motion, we recommend performing static (non-ballistic) stretching or flexibility training after a 4–5-minute warm-up period or after an aerobic or strength training routine to reduce the risk of muscle injury and pain. In a clinical population, if aerobic training and strength training occur on the same day, the best approach is to perform the activity that is the primary training focus of that day first (Ehrman et al., 2023).

A comprehensive exercise prescription should consider each person's specific goals. Common objectives include the following:
- Improve appearance
- Improve the quality of life
- Manage weight

- Preparation for the competition
- Improve overall health to reduce the risk of primary or secondary onset of disease
- Reduce the burden of a chronic disease or condition (early fatigue, depression, loss of personal control, economic impact) (Ehrman et al., 2023).

People with specific diseases often have goals directly related to reversing or reducing the progression of the disease and its side effects or the side effects of therapies used to treat the disorder. A kinesiologist must have a complete understanding of how to modify the overall exercise prescription in order to provide the patient with the best chance of success in achieving the desired goal. Furthermore, it should help evaluate whether goals are realistic and discuss them with patients when they are not (Ehrman et al., 2023).

Basic training principles apply to all types of exercise programs, whether the goal is to improve cardiorespiratory fitness, musculoskeletal fitness, body composition, or flexibility. The principles of training are as follows:

- *Specificity-of-training principle*

  The principle of specificity states that the body's physiological and metabolic responses and adaptations to training are specific to the type of exercise and muscle

groups involved. For example, motor activities that require continuous, dynamic and rhythmic contractions of large muscle groups are more suitable for stimulating improvements in cardiorespiratory endurance; stretching exercises develop joint range of motion and flexibility; and resistance exercises are effective for improving muscle strength and muscular endurance. Furthermore, gains in muscle efficiency depend on the muscle groups trained, the type and speed of contraction, and the intensity of training (Gibson et al., 2024).

- *Overload training principle*

    To encourage the improvement of the components of physical fitness it is necessary to accustom the body's physiological systems by using greater loads (principle of overload) than those to which the individual is accustomed. As individuals approach their genetic ceiling, the rate of improvement in physical fitness slows and eventually levels off (principle of diminishing returns). Overload can be achieved by increasing the frequency, intensity and duration of aerobic exercise. Muscle groups can be effectively overloaded by increasing the number of repetitions, sets, or exercises in programs that improve muscle fitness and flexibility (Gibson et al., 2024).

- *Principle of progression*

  Throughout your training program, you need to progressively increase your training volume, or overload, to stimulate further improvements. Progression must be gradual because doing too much too soon can cause musculoskeletal injuries (Gibson et al., 2024).

- *Principle of initial values*

  Individuals with low initial levels of physical fitness will show greater relative gains (%) and a faster rate of improvement in response to training than individuals with medium or high levels of physical fitness (baseline principle). For example, during the first month of an aerobic exercise program, the VO_2 max of an individual with poor cardiorespiratory endurance capacity may improve by 12% or more, while a highly trained endurance athlete may improve by only 1% or less. This is one of the main reasons why some individuals abandon training programs (Gibson et al., 2024).

- *Principle of interindividual variability*

  Individual responses to a training stimulus are quite variable and depend on a series of factors such as age, initial physical fitness level and state of health (principle of interindividual variability). It is therefore necessary to design exercise programs with the specific needs, interests, and abilities of each client in mind and to develop personalized exercise prescriptions that take into account individual differences and preferences (Gibson et al., 2024).

- *Principle of diminishing returns*
  Each person has a genetic ceiling that limits the amount of improvement possible with physical training. As individuals approach their genetic ceiling, the rate of improvement in physical fitness slows and eventually plateaus (Gibson et al., 2024).

- *Principle of reversibility*
  The positive physiological effects and health benefits of regular physical activity and exercise are reversible. When individuals stop exercise programs (detraining), exercise capacity declines rapidly. Within a few months, most training improvements are lost (Gibson et al., 2024).

Since fibromyalgia (FM) is classified as a chronic non-communicable disease, the same recommendations and principles, mentioned previously, can be used for the treatment of this syndrome.

There is considerable evidence to support the use of exercise as a cornerstone in the management of FM (Burckhardt et al., 1994).

This research shows that both aerobic exercise and strength training can reduce the severity of many symptoms associated with FM, including pain levels, fatigue, depression, and sleep disturbances (Bircan et al., 2008). Since obesity and overweight are common in people with FM, weight control has also proven to be an effective tool in reducing symptoms (Rossi et al., 2015). People with FM often have a very narrow therapeutic window for physical activity due to the high levels of pain and stiffness associated with this disorder. Additionally, exercise is often an aggravator of symptoms. For this reason, many people with FM avoid physical activity, fearing that their symptoms will intensify. As a result, most individuals with FM remain aerobically inactive, with poor muscle strength and limited flexibility (Jones & Clark, 2002). Therefore, training programs for this population should emphasize increasing functional activity levels without causing post-exertional pain and fatigue.

Gradually accumulating at least 5,000 steps per day can lead to clinically significant reductions in pain intensity (Kaleth et al., 2014).

Post-exercise disorders are typically found in strength and conditioning programs that use high-intensity, higher-impact movements and fail to allow patients to self-regulate exercise intensity (Jones et al., 2006). Therefore, light to moderate intensity exercise performed all or most days of the week is recommended.

Additionally, because the severity of symptoms can vary greatly daily, the kinesiologist must be able to manipulate the volume, intensity, and duration of exercise based on pain tolerance and acute attacks of fatigue. It would be advisable to assess the severity of the patient's symptoms before physical activity.

Resistance training can be beneficial to those with FM by helping to improve isometric and dynamic muscle strength, as well as power (Hakkinen et al., 2001).

By improving strength and power, FM patients may be able to perform activities of daily living with greater ease, thus conserving energy and minimizing the effects of fatigue. It is recommended that the kinesiologist initially choose at least one exercise for each of the major muscle groups in order to promote overall muscle development (Gavi et al., 2014). If during the use of any of the selected exercises or in the days following training a musculoskeletal worsening occurs, the exercises used could be modified or replaced with others that are more bearable. Start with two training sessions per week with at least three days between sessions and a conservative training frequency. As patients' functional abilities and tolerance improve, they can progress to three training sessions per week with at least 48 hours between sessions. Some people with FM may actually better tolerate a four-day-per-week routine in which different muscle groups are trained on different days. This reduces the intensity of each individual workout by dispersing the workload and volume typically performed across two training days over four days. It may also be helpful to intermittently incorporate cardiovascular and flexibility exercises between sets to provide clients with the opportunity to rest between strength training exercises, thus improving exercise tolerance while still using their time effectively (Duncan & Achara, 2003).

Selecting the appropriate intensity level for FM sufferers is often a process of trial and error that requires the kinesiologist to select an appropriate training load to elicit positive adaptation without creating significant increases in pain or discomfort. Patients should start by performing at least one set of 10 to 15 repetitions and gradually increase training volume as tolerance improves and tension levels increase. Once the patient can perform 12 to 15 repetitions with correct form and without excessive pain and fatigue, the amount of resistance can be progressively increased with initial reductions in volume (Kraemer et al., 2018).

Therefore, the number of repetitions performed should initially decrease as the training load increases to help prevent excessive microtrauma.

Daily cardiorespiratory exercise should be encouraged. Typically, low-impact, light-intensity aerobic exercises such as walking, cycling, or water aerobic activity in a heated pool are generally well tolerated by the FM population (Jones & Clark, 2002). Additionally, because repetitive movements tend to aggravate FM symptoms, some people can tolerate shorter exercise intervals of 5 to 10 minutes throughout the day instead of one long exercise session. It is recommended to start with a light intensity for 10 to 15 minutes twice a day and to increase the duration of activity to 30 to 40 minutes three to four days a week as tolerated (LaFontaine, 2000).

Performing passive, slow static stretching intermittently during exercise sessions can also improve a patient's tolerance to exercise by allowing clients the opportunity to rest between exercises. Stretching at regular intervals throughout the day can also help reduce pain and stiffness and improve mobility and can help prevent muscle pain and stiffness after remaining in one position for a long period. Initially, the individual should attempt to hold each stretch for approximately 10 to 15 seconds or if tolerance allows. As tolerance improves, the duration of each stretch can vary progressively, increasing up to 20-30 seconds. Although each stretch can be held for a longer duration, stretching longer than 30 seconds may be too intense and increase discomfort. Therefore, it may be helpful to stretch more frequently rather than for longer periods.

Additionally, daily stretching can help manage the muscle soreness and stiffness often experienced by these clients.

Stretching intensity should remain relatively low with an emphasis on stretching only to the point where the muscles feel tight, never to the threshold of pain or tenderness. This is an important consideration as overstretching can increase the likelihood of microtrauma in muscle tissues along with increased pain and stiffness (Kraemer et al., 2018).

What has been said regarding the different types of training leads us to identify the *multicomponent exercise* as the most effective as it is able to include them all in a single training session. Multicomponent training could offer unique benefits beyond a single exercise intervention, as individuals may benefit from effects associated with multiple forms of exercise (aerobic, strength, flexibility) that offer the potential to train the cardiorespiratory systems, vascular and neuromusculoskeletal (Garber et al., 2011).

Physical exercise for fibromyalgia patients presents recommendations and contraindications for training which are the following:

1. Be prepared for the fact that progress in all health-related components of physical fitness will take much longer than that in apparently healthy individuals.

2. Kinesiologists should be aware of how subjects respond to training and be willing to adjust frequency, intensity, and time as needed. Avoiding painful movements is vital to this process.

3. Aerobic training should be light and low impact at first.

4. Strength training can include many different modalities but should begin with low-intensity activities until tolerance can be determined. Consider bodyweight activities, low-intensity strength

training modalities such as tubes and bands, and movements with machines and free weights.

5. Avoid ballistic movements during training. Use smooth, controlled movements that will reduce the risk of injury and allow adequate control of movements.

6. Initially consider aerobic modalities which are predictable modes of exercise so that the client can exercise more effectively in a sedentary state.

7. Consider alternating low-intensity static stretching between strength training sets.

8. Alternative modes of exercise are also useful. Consider water exercises, Qi Gong, or meditation (Kraemer et al., 2018).

Exercise professionals need to know the ideal and specific dosage to administer exercise to everyone. Although the positive effects of exercise are well known for addressing common symptoms and comorbidities in people with FM, there is an urgent need for further investigation into exercise dosing about FITT-VP principles (frequency, intensity, time, type, volume, and progression) according to the American College of Sports Medicine guidelines (2017). This need becomes central because FM patients have a very low rate of adherence to physical exercise (Schmidt-Wilcke & Clauw, 2011); this occurs not only due to the exacerbation of symptoms but also due to the contradictory information regarding exercise that these patients receive from the professionals who are part of their treatment group (Rooks, 2008).

Therefore, paragraph 5.2 will propose the methods of physical exercise present in the most recent scientific literature to improve the psychophysical well-being of subjects suffering from FM, highlighting the ideal dosages of exercise in relation to the FITT-VP principles.

Finally, in paragraph 5.3 an example of a multicomponent physical exercise protocol adapted to subjects with FM will be presented.

5.2 Exercise dosage in relation to FITT-VP training principles

The American College of Sports Medicine has proposed the acronym FITT-VP (Frequency, Intensity, Time, Type, Volume, and Progression) which represents a valid guide for exercise prescription. Correctly modulating frequency, intensity, time, type, volume, and progression represents the key to transforming physical activity into an exercise with precise therapeutic and functional objectives (ACSM, 2017); in fact, it is considered a real principle (FITT-VP Principle) on which the programming of an adapted physical exercise program must be based, as is the case for FM.

FM is currently treated with both pharmacological and non-pharmacological means (Rossy et al., 1999); physical exercise has found wide application in the clinical field (Thompson et al., 2013) and is considered the non-pharmacological approach par excellence to the treatment of this pathology (Kelley et al., 2011). In fact, several studies confirm how different types of exercise (for example aerobic, strength, flexibility) contribute positively to the quality of life of subjects with FM, improving the negative symptoms related to this syndrome (Andrade et al., 2020).

However, there is a need to further investigate exercise dosing in relation to FITT-VP parameters. For this reason, we took care of evaluating what the scientific literature provides regarding the effects of physical activity with respect to FM, trying to identify the best training protocol and the most effective FITT-VP parameters.

5.2.1 Frequency

The first parameter taken into consideration is frequency which generally refers to the total number of training sessions per week; it is related to the duration and intensity of exercise and varies depending on the client's program goals and preferences, time constraints, and functional capacity (ACSM, 2017).

About FM, in the different studies taken into consideration, the frequency may differ based on the protocol used, specifically, it is recommended to perform strength exercises 2 to 3 days a week, aerobic exercises 2 to 4 days a week, and of flexibility from 1 to 3 days a week to attenuate or reduce signs and symptoms (Pescatello, 2014).

The ideal would be to start with two weekly workouts and progress up to four as the weeks go by, trying to combine the different protocols in these sessions (i.e., multicomponent protocol).

5.2.2 Intensity

Exercise or physical activity intensity refers to the objectively measured work or subjectively determined level of effort performed by an individual (ACSM, 2017).

Typical objective measures of work that are important to the kinesiologist include heart rate, oxygen consumption (VO_2max or MET), caloric expenditure (kilocalories [kcal] or joule [J]), mass or weight lifted (kilograms), and the power output (watts [W]).

The subjective level of effort can be assessed through a verbal statement from the person performing the exercise (for example, "I'm tired" or "It's easy"), the so-called talk test (i.e., the fastest possible pace while still able to carry on a conversation) or a standardized scale (for example, the Borg rating of perceived effort). As regards the Borg scale, it is necessary to teach the patient the correct use of this assessment tool to obtain precise indications of perceived effort (Ehrman et al., 2023).

Individuals with FM may have problems adapting to physical exercise due to soreness, fatigue, and soreness after exercise (Bidonde et al., 2014), also for this reason, the intensity of exercise for these subjects must be between light and moderate (aerobic activity with a range between 60/65% of HRmax; strength exercises with a load between 30% and 60% of 1 repetition maximum (1RM) (Sousa et al., 2023).

5.2.3 Time

Duration (or time, the first T of the acronym FITT) refers to the amount of time spent engaging in exercise or physical activity (ACSM, 2017).

Exercise duration and intensity are inversely related: the higher the intensity, the shorter the duration of exercise. The duration of exercise depends not only on the intensity of the exercise but also on the patient's health status, initial fitness level, functional capacity, and program goals. To improve health benefits, it is recommended that individuals with FM accumulate at least 150 minutes of moderate-intensity physical activity per week (ACSM, 2017).

This amount of physical activity can be achieved either in continuous daily periods (e.g., 45/60 minutes of moderate-intensity effort for 2-4 days/week) depending on the client's functional capacity and time constraints (ACSM, 2017).

As the client adapts to training, exercise duration can be slowly increased (e.g., by 5 to 10 minutes per session) approximately every 1 to 2 weeks for at least the first month. For older and less fit individuals, the ACSM (2017) recommends increasing exercise duration, rather than intensity, early in the exercise program;

however, gradually moving the patient towards the minimum required threshold of both duration and intensity is important in terms of maximizing the benefits of the program. For most patients, the duration of aerobic, strength, and flexibility training should not exceed 60 minutes. This will reduce the possibility of overuse injuries and exercise burnout (ACSM, 2017).

From the studies present in the literature it can be deduced that the optimal duration of each training session to obtain an improvement in each parameter evaluated in subjects affected by FM is between 60 and 90 minutes, with training protocols lasting longer than 6 weeks which they appear to have the best effects in patients.

5.2.4 Type

The second T of the acronym FITT-VP refers to the type and method of execution of the exercise; individuals with FM may have different responses to different types of exercise protocols: aerobic, strength, flexibility, aquatic, pilates, tai chi (Kolak et al., 2022).

These protocols are used in the literature both individually and in association with each other; for example, the coupling of aerobic exercise with other exercise modalities is fundamental as it induces adaptations in different systems, in particular the cardiovascular, energetic, neuromuscular and neuroendocrine systems (Bidonde et al., 1996); the latter allows an increase in serotonin and norepinephrine concentrations, with a consequent improvement in mood and greater psychophysical well-being (Busch et al., 2008).

Since these individuals present a great diversity of signs and symptoms, multicomponent exercise protocols should be preferred that are able to provide positive effects on a greater number of symptoms (Neira et al., 2024), but not only, as they represent the set of all the protocols previously mentioned in a single training session; in fact, multicomponent training is defined as a form of training that involves the combined execution of a variety of exercises to develop strength, balance, flexibility and cardiovascular resistance all in a single training session (López-López et al., 2023).

5.2.5 Volume and Progression

Volume is the total amount of exercise necessary to obtain a result while progression is how training parameters are modified, to continue improvements or to adapt to the needs of the person (ACSM, 2017).

For the improvement of signs and symptoms related to FM, in relation to the volume and progression parameters, it is recommended to start with an initial volume between 8-12 repetitions and progress up to 15-20, associating them with an initial number of sets of 2 per then move on to 4 sets of each exercise.

5.3 Example of an exercise protocol adapted to subjects with Fibromyalgia

From the previous paragraph, the multicomponent protocol is the most appropriate type of physical exercise for subjects suffering from FM.

In this paragraph, we have reported an example of an adapted multicomponent physical exercise protocol for which the literature has demonstrated its effectiveness in improving physical fitness and quality of life in patients suffering from FM.

Table 5.1 shows a multicomponent physical exercise protocol to be carried out in the initial phase, while Table 5.2 shows the central phase of an advanced multicomponent exercise protocol to be carried out after approximately 4-6 weeks of physical activity. By scanning the QR Codes it is possible to consult the online videos showing the execution of the exercises.

Table 5.1 Example of a multicomponent exercise protocol to be carried out in the initial phase.

WARM-UP		
	WALK IN PLACE Duration: 120 seconds Walk in place at a moderate speed. Place your entire foot on the ground and alternately lift your knees.	

RETRACTION OF THE SCAPULAES

20 Repetitions
Grasp a stick with both hands and extend your arms in front. Bring your shoulders forward and back while keeping your arms extended and feel the moving away and coming together of your shoulder blades respectively. Keep the lumbar curve neutral and stable.

ARMS RAISE WITH STICK

10 repetitions
Grasp a stick with both hands. Bring the stick above your head while keeping your arms extended. Maintain the lumbar curve.

ARMS RAISE WITH STICK (BOUNCE)

10 repetitions
Grasp a stick with both hands. Bring the stick above your head while keeping your arms extended and perform a small bounce once you reach maximum joint excursion. Maintain the lumbar curve.

HIP ROTATION

10 repetitions per side
Maintain balance on one foot, using the cane (or other supports). Perform the external and internal rotation movement of the hip slowly and maintaining the lumbar curve.

CENTRAL PHASE

WALK IN PLACE

Duration: 30 seconds
Recovery: 30 seconds
Walk in place at a moderate speed. Place your entire foot on the ground and alternately lift your knees.

SIDEWALK

Duration: 30 seconds
Recovery: 30 seconds
Lateral walking Be careful to maintain balance when moving sideways.

	BENDING ON THE LEGS (SQUAT) 10 repetitions Recovery: 60 seconds Place your feet shoulder-width apart. Keeping your body weight over the center of your feet, bend your knees until you feel an activation in the front of your thigh. Be careful to maintain the physiological curves of your back.	
	HIP FLEXION AND ARMS EXTENSION 10 reps per leg Recovery: 60 seconds Raise both arms above your head and knees alternately. Be careful to keep your balance on the supporting foot and pull up the toe that comes off the ground.	
	HEEL RAISING 10 repetitions Recovery: 45 seconds From a standing position, lift your heels quickly and descend in a controlled manner. Between reps, don't let your heels touch the floor. If necessary, help yourself with support to maintain balance.	

GLUTE BRIDGE

10 repetitions
Recovery: 45 seconds
Lie on your stomach, flex your legs, placing your feet hip-width apart and as close to your buttocks as possible. From this position, lift your pelvis, trying to bring your shoulders, pelvis and knees on the same imaginary line. Descend in a controlled manner.

QUADRUPED EXERCISE

10 reps per side
Recovery: 60 seconds
In the quadruped position, lower the upper limb and the contralateral lower limb at the same time. During the execution of the movement, maintain the physiological curves and keep the pelvis parallel to the ground.

DONKEY KICKS

10 reps per side
Recovery: 60 seconds
In a quadruped position, place your hands under your shoulders and your knees under your hips. Raise one leg imagining you must touch the ceiling with your foot.
Check your pelvis to keep it parallel to the ground and not arch your back. Return in a controlled manner.

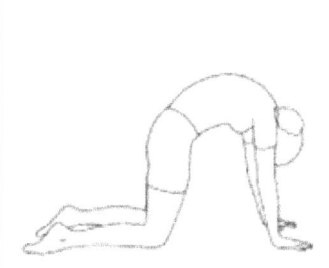	**CURL DUMBBELLS** 10 repetitions Recovery: 45 seconds In a standing position, flex your elbows at the same time, bringing the dumbbells towards the shoulder of the same arm. If you don't have dumbbells, use water bottles or other household tools.	
COOL DOWN – 20 second pause between exercises		
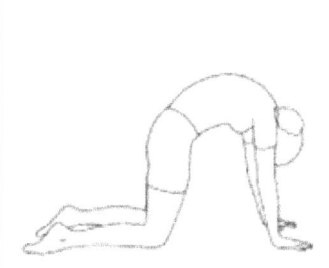	**CAT-COW** 12 Repetitions Assume a quadruped position with hands under shoulders and knees under hips. Pelvis in retroversion and push with your hands to make the "hump" and flex the head. Pelvis in anteversion, arch your back with straight arms and extend your head. inhale with your head up and exhale with your head down.	
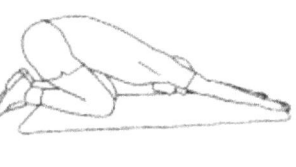	**CHILD POSE** 3 times for 30 Seconds From a quadruped position, bring your buttocks to your heels by stretching your hands until you feel a stretch at the dorsal level.	

	QUADRICEPS STRETCH	
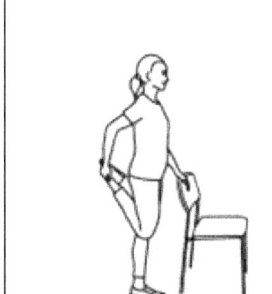	2 repetitions for 30 seconds per side From a standing position, grasp the foot with your hand, bending the knee until you feel a stretching sensation in the front part of the thigh. If necessary, use a support to maintain balance	

It is advisable to use the previous protocol for the initial phases of training (approximately 4/6 weeks) and subsequently implement it with the protocol shown in table 5.2 to respect the FITT-VP principles previously illustrated; specifically, the methods of execution of some exercises will vary, the intensity of the aerobic component will also change entirely and some exercises will also change entirely and be replaced with others, deemed more valid and effective following the increase in the level of training of the subjects.

Table 5.2 Central phase of an advanced multicomponent exercise protocol to be carried out after 4/6 weeks.

CENTRAL PHASE		
	WALK IN PLACE Duration: 30 seconds. Recovery: 30 seconds. Walk in place at a moderate speed. Place your entire foot on the ground and alternately lift your knees.	

LATERAL WALK WITH UPPER LIMBS

Duration: 30 seconds
Recovery: 30 seconds
Lateral walk with overhead movement of the arms. Bring your arms up as I move my feet apart and bring them back down when they come together again. Be careful to maintain balance and control movement.

BENDING ON THE LEGS WITH UPPER LIMBS

10 repetitions
Recovery: 60 seconds
Place your feet shoulder-width apart. Keeping your body weight over the center of your feet, bend your knees until you feel an activation in the front of your thigh. When ascending, raise one arm alternately above your head

FRONT LUNGES

8 repetitions per leg
Recovery: 60 seconds
From a standing position, take a step back and keep your body weight distributed on both feet. Bend both knees and try to bring the back knee as close to the floor as possible, without touching it. Push with both legs and return to the starting position

SIDE LUNGES

8 reps per leg
Recovery: 60 seconds
From a standing position, take a sidestep and shift your body weight onto the moving foot. Fold the_knee and keep the remaining leg straight. Push with the bent leg and return to the starting position

HEEL RAISING

10 repetitions
Recovery: 45 seconds
From a standing position, lift your heels quickly and descend in a controlled manner. Between reps, don't let your heels touch the floor.
If necessary, help yourself with support to maintain balance.

GLUTE BRIDGE

10 repetitions
Recovery: 45 seconds
Lie on your stomach, flex your legs, placing your feet hip-width apart and as close to your buttocks as possible. From this position, lift your pelvis, trying to bring your shoulders, pelvis and knees on the same imaginary line. Descend in a controlled manner.

QUADRUPED EXERCISE

10 repetitions per side
Recovery: 60 seconds
In the quadruped position, extend the contralateral upper limb and lower limb at the same time. During the execution of the movement, maintain the physiological curves and keep the pelvis parallel to the ground.

DONKEY KICKS

10 repetitions per side
Recovery: 60 seconds
In a quadruped position, place your hands under your shoulders and your knees under your hips. Raise one leg imagining you must touch the ceiling with your foot.
Check your pelvis to keep it parallel to the ground and not arch your back. Return in a controlled manner.

CURL DUMBBELLS

10 repetitions
Recovery: 45 seconds
In a standing position, flex your elbows at the same time, bringing the dumbbells towards the shoulder of the same arm.
If you don't have dumbbells, use water bottles or other household tools.

References

American College of Sports Medicine. (2017). *ACSM's Guidelines for Exercise Testing and Prescription*. 10th ed. New York: Wolters Kluwer.

Andrade, A., Dominski, F. H., & Sieczkowska, S. M. (2020, December). What we already know about the effects of exercise in patients with fibromyalgia: An umbrella review. In *Seminars in arthritis and rheumatism* (Vol. 50, No. 6, pp. 1465-1480). WB Saunders.

Bidonde, J., Busch, A. J., Schachter, C. L., Overend, T. J., Kim, S. Y., Góes, S. M., ... & Cochrane Musculoskeletal Group. (1996). Aerobic exercise training for adults with fibromyalgia. *Cochrane Database of Systematic Reviews, 2017*(6).

Bidonde, J., Jean Busch, A., Bath, B., & Milosavljevic, S. (2014). Exercise for adults with fibromyalgia: an umbrella systematic review with synthesis of best evidence. *Current rheumatology reviews, 10*(1), 45-79.

Bircan, Ç., Karasel, S. A., Akgün, B., El, Ö., & Alper, S. (2008). Effects of muscle strengthening versus aerobic exercise program in fibromyalgia. *Rheumatology international, 28*, 527-532.

Bull, F. C., Al-Ansari, S. S., Biddle, S., Borodulin, K., Buman, M. P., Cardon, G., ... & Willumsen, J. F. (2020). World Health Organization 2020 guidelines on physical activity and sedentary behaviour. *British Journal of Sports Medicine, 54*(24), 1451-1462.

Burckhardt, C. S., Mannerkorpi, K., Hedenberg, L., & Bjelle, A. (1994). A randomized, controlled clinical trial of education and physical training for women with fibromyalgia. *The Journal of Rheumatology, 21*(4), 714-720.

Busch, A. J., Schachter, C. L., Overend, T. J., Peloso, P. M., & Barber, K. A. (2008). Exercise for fibromyalgia: a systematic review. *The Journal of rheumatology, 35*(6), 1130-1144.

Coombes, J. S., Law, J., Lancashire, B., & Fassett, R. G. (2015). "Exercise is medicine" curbing the burden of chronic disease and physical inactivity. *Asia Pacific Journal of Public Health, 27*(2), NP600-NP605.

DECRETO LEGISLATIVO 28 febbraio 2021, n. 36. https://www.gazzettaufficiale.it/eli/id/2021/03/18/21G00043/sg

Duncan, H. V., & Achara, G. (2003). A rare initial manifestation of systemic lupus erythematosus—acute pancreatitis: case report and review of the literature. *The Journal of the American Board of Family Practice*, *16*(4), 334-338.

Ehrman, J. K., Gordon, P. M., Visich, P. S., & Keteyian, S. J. (Eds.). (2023). *Clinical exercise physiology: exercise management for chronic diseases and special populations*. Human Kinetics.

Eijsvogels, T. M., & Thompson, P. D. (2015). Exercise is medicine: at any dose?. *Jama*, *314*(18), 1915-1916.

Farinella, A., Mosso, C. O., & Leonardi, D. (2016). Attività motoria e sportiva come strategia per promuovere l'inclusione: una prospettiva dell'attività fisica adattata. *Formazione & insegnamento*, *14*(3 Suppl.), 85-92.

Garber, C. E., Blissmer, B., Deschenes, M. R., Franklin, B. A., Lamonte, M. J., Lee, I. M., ... & Swain, D. P. (2011). Quantity and quality of exercise for developing and maintaining cardiorespiratory, musculoskeletal, and neuromotor fitness in apparently healthy adults: guidance for prescribing exercise. *Medicine & science in sports & exercise*, *43*(7), 1334-1359.

Gavi, M. B. R. O., Vassalo, D. V., Amaral, F. T., Macedo, D. C. F., Gava, P. L., Dantas, E. M., & Valim, V. (2014). Strengthening exercises improve symptoms and quality of life but do not change autonomic modulation in fibromyalgia: a randomized clinical trial. *PloS one*, *9*(3), e90767.

Gibson, A. L., Wagner, D. R., & Heyward, V. H. (2024). *Advanced fitness assessment and exercise prescription*. Human kinetics.

Häkkinen, A., Häkkinen, K., Hannonen, P., & Alen, M. (2001). Strength training induced adaptations in neuromuscular function of premenopausal women with fibromyalgia: comparison with healthy women. *Annals of the rheumatic diseases*, *60*(1), 21-26.

Jones, K. D., & Clark, S. R. (2002). Individualizing the exercise prescription for persons with fibromyalgia. *Rheumatic Disease Clinics*, *28*(2), 419-436.

Jones, K. D., Adams, D., Winters-Stone, K., & Burckhardt, C. S. (2006). A comprehensive review of 46 exercise treatment studies in fibromyalgia (1988–2005). *Health and quality of life outcomes*, *4*, 1-6.

Kaleth, A. S., Slaven, J. E., & Ang, D. C. (2014). Does increasing steps per day predict improvement in physical function and pain interference in adults with fibromyalgia?. *Arthritis care & research*, *66*(12), 1887-1894.

Kelley, G. A., & Kelley, K. S. (2011). Exercise improves global well-being in adults with fibromyalgia: confirmation of previous meta-analytic results using a recently developed and novel varying coefficient model. *Clinical and Experimental Rheumatology-Incl Supplements*, *29*(6), S60.

Kolak, E., Ardıç, F., & Fındıkoğlu, G. (2022). Effects of different types of exercises on pain, quality of life, depression, and body composition in women with fibromyalgia: A three-arm, parallel-group, randomized trial. *Archives of Rheumatology*, *37*(3), 444.

Kraemer, W. J., Comstock, B. A., & Clark, J. E. (2018). NSCA's Essentials of Training Special Populations. *Champaign, IL: Human Kinetics*.

LaFontaine, T. (2000). Special populations. *Strength and Conditioning Journal*, *22*(5), 42-44.

López-López, S., Abuín-Porras, V., Berlanga, L. A., Martos-Duarte, M., Perea-Unceta, L., Romero-Morales, C., & Pareja-Galeano, H. (2023). Functional mobility and physical fitness are improved through a multicomponent training program in institutionalized older adults. *GeroScience*, *46*(1), 1201–1209. https://doi.org/10.1007/s11357-023-00877-4

Lundqvist, S., Börjesson, M., Larsson, M. E., Hagberg, L., & Cider, Å. (2017). Physical Activity on Prescription (PAP), in patients with metabolic risk factors. A 6-month follow-up study in primary health care. *PLoS One*, *12*(4), e0175190.

Martin, D., Carl, K., & Lehnertz, K. (1997). *Manuale di teoria dell'allenamento*. Società stampa sportiva.

Neira, S. R., Marques, A. P., Cervantes, R. F., Pillado, M. S., & Costa, J. V. (2024). Efficacy of aquatic vs land-based therapy for pain management in women with fibromyalgia: a randomised controlled trial. *Physiotherapy*, *123*, 91-101.

Pescatello, L. S. (Ed.). (2014). *ACSM's guidelines for exercise testing and prescription*. Lippincott Williams & Wilkins.

Pescatello, L. S., Franklin, B. A., Fagard, R., Farquhar, W. B., Kelley, G. A., & Ray, C. A. (2004). Exercise and hypertension. *Medicine & science in sports & exercise*, *36*(3), 533-553.

Rooks, D. S. (2008). Talking to patients with fibromyalgia about physical activity and exercise. *Current opinion in Rheumatology*, *20*(2), 208-212.

Rossi, A., Di Lollo, A. C., Guzzo, M. P., Giacomelli, C., Atzeni, F., Bazzichi, L., & Di Franco, M. (2015). Fibromyalgia and nutrition: what news. *Clin Exp Rheumatol*, *33*(1 Suppl 88), S117-25.

Rossy, L. A., Buckelew, S. P., Dorr, N., Hagglund, K. J., Thayer, J. F., McIntosh, M. J., ... & Johnson, J. C. (1999). A meta-analysis of fibromyalgia treatment interventions. *Annals of behavioral medicine*, *21*(2), 180-191.

Same, R. V., Feldman, D. I., Shah, N., Martin, S. S., Al Rifai, M., Blaha, M. J., ... & Ahmed, H. M. (2016). Relationship between sedentary behavior and cardiovascular risk. *Current cardiology reports*, *18*, 1-7.

Schmidt-Wilcke, T., & Clauw, D. J. (2011). Fibromyalgia: from pathophysiology to therapy. *Nature Reviews Rheumatology*, *7*(9), 518-527.

Sousa, M., et al. (2023, June). Effects of combined training programs in individuals with fibromyalgia: a systematic review. *In Healthcare* (Vol. 11, No. 12, p. 1708). MDPI.

Thompson, P. D., Arena, R., Riebe, D., & Pescatello, L. S. (2013). ACSM's new preparticipation health screening recommendations from ACSM's guidelines for exercise testing and prescription. *Current sports medicine reports*, *12*(4), 215-217.

US Department of Health and Human Services. (2008). US Department of Health and Human Services 2008 physical activity guidelines for Americans. *Hyattsville, MD: Author, Washington, DC*, *2008*, 1-40.

Wen, C. P., Wai, J. P. M., Tsai, M. K., Yang, Y. C., Cheng, T. Y. D., Lee, M. C., ... & Wu, X. (2011). Minimum amount of physical activity for reduced mortality and extended life expectancy: a prospective cohort study. *The lancet, 378*(9798), 1244-1253.

Word Health Organization (2020). WHO guidelines on physical activity and sedentary behaviour. Geneva: World Health Organization. www.who.int/publications/i/item/9789240015128

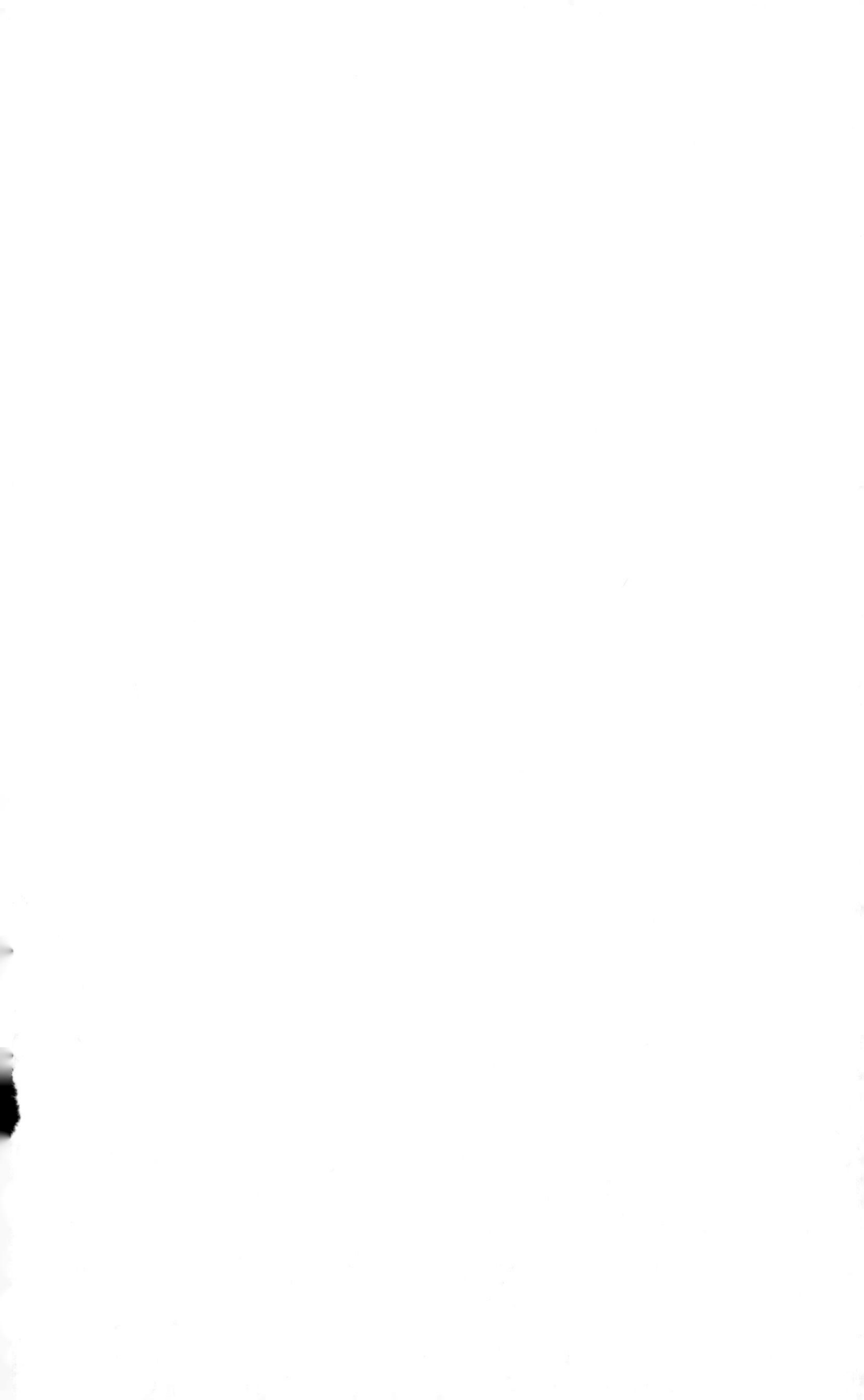

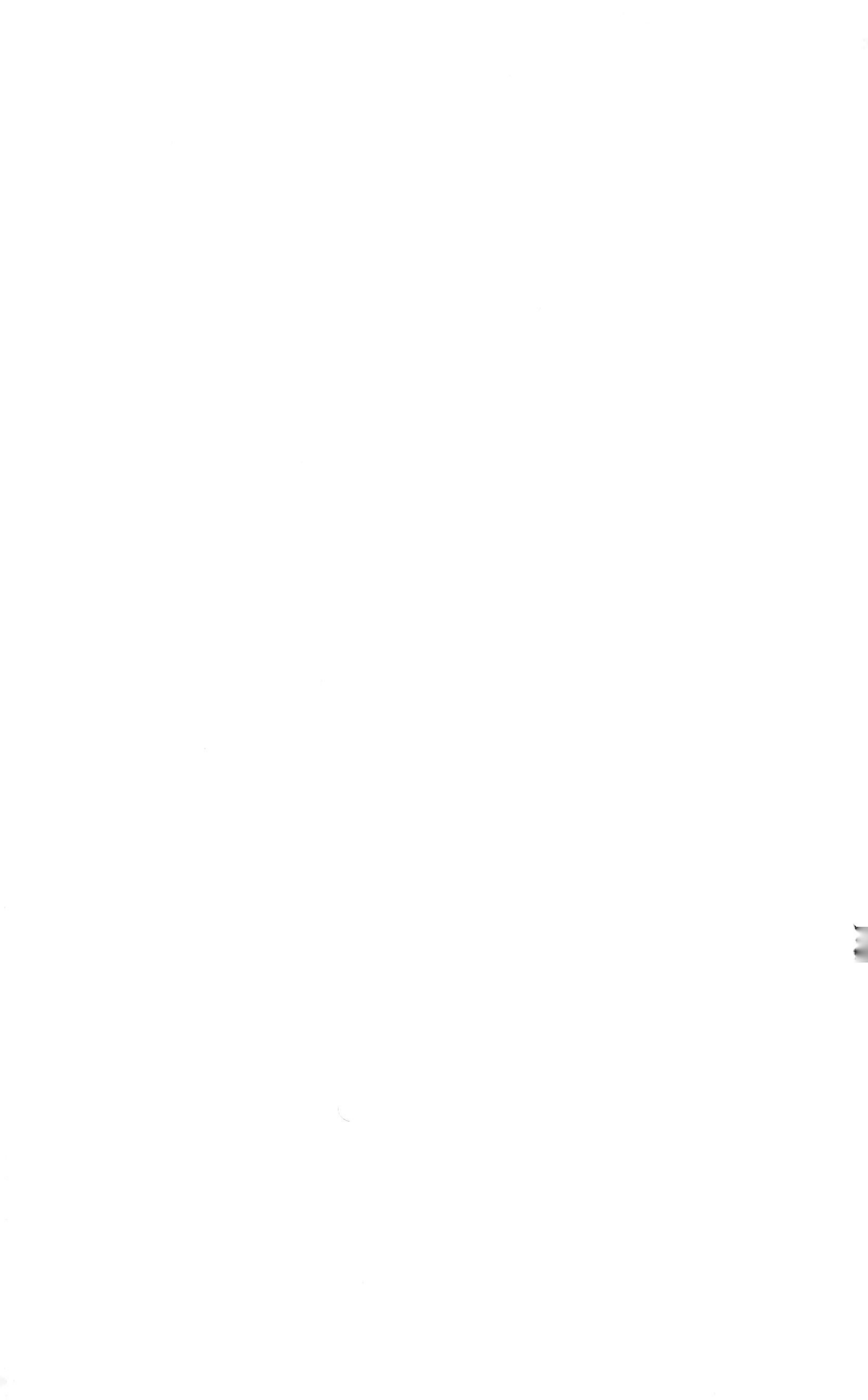

www.ingramcontent.com/pod-product-compliance
Lightning Source LLC
Chambersburg PA
CBHW052147220526
45471CB00004B/1567